thenickelallergycookbook@yahoo.com

ISBN 9798847535915

First Book Edition 2016

Cream Cheese Drops used by permission from LorAnn Gourmet Foods

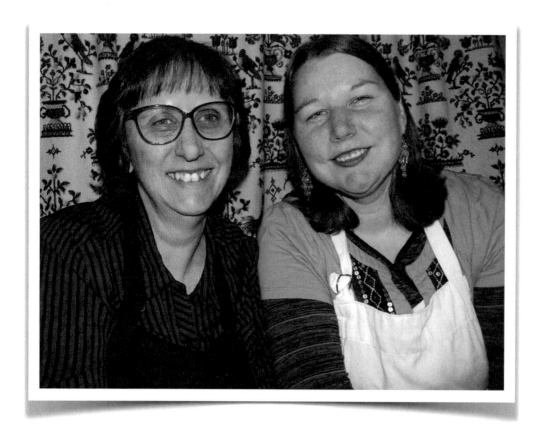

Judy Bratz (left) and Charity Bratz (right)

This book is dedicated to all the moms who had to hold the hand of their loved one in the E.R. while they had an allergic reaction, not knowing if they were going to live or die.

Judy Bratz

This book is dedicated to my family, friends, and all those who struggle with nickel allergies.

Charity Bratz

Table of Contents

Preface

In this cookbook are recipes my mother and I have made and modified to accommodate a low nickel diet. We are not doctors, specialists, or prestigious chefs, but I am a patient.

We developed this book when we found out I had a severe nickel allergy and would have to make some major changes to my diet in order to live. I am into my eleventh year of managing my allergies and have survived thirteen near-death emergency room visits. It took eight of those years to determine that the various foods I was eating were causing my tongue and throat swelling, my stomach ailments, headaches, nasal allergies, and a chronically low immune system.

The root of my allergies was difficult to determine since I reacted to so many different foods, it seemed, without a causal link. It wasn't until my tenth reaction on my birthday at a Chinese restaurant that found us looking for alternatives with an allergist. After numerous skin tests, we discovered that the causal link was my reaction to nickel in the foods I ate. All of the foods had been high in nickel content and, when added together, caused a severe allergic reaction.

Overjoyed, I thought my worries were over! I would have a list I could stick to so I wouldn't have any more reactions. Of course, things are never that simple. I clutched the meager list of forty foods I had received from the doctor, and I was crestfallen at the limitations of my diet. I had to find a way to expand it.

I searched online for hours, finding nothing but contradictory information, until I stumbled upon a study conducted by the FDA on 300 foods and their nickel levels. I cross-referenced it with the list the doctor gave me to determine my range of what was good to eat, what I could have in moderation, and what I had to avoid at all costs. From there, making adjustments to the list was just trial and error.

With a more complete list in hand, I spent hours in the store reading labels and buying groceries. I was surprised at how many foods were high in nickel, and disappointed when they were foods I liked and used frequently. I had to find alternatives if I ever wanted to eat normally.

Some of the foods I could eat were unfamiliar to both my mother and I. We poured over cookbooks to find recipes I could modify and make work. We finally had to resign ourselves to making our own recipes because there just wasn't a cookbook out there for nickel sufferers. Now we can say there is.

Nickel Allergies

What is it?

Nickel allergies occur when the body reacts to the presence of a foreign object, namely nickel, in an effort to purge it from the system. Nasal passages inflame, exposed body parts swell or rash, skin burns or blisters, and the immune system rushes to attack the intrusion like a disease. The most noticeable and common reactions are external — to jewelry, pant buttons, belt buckles, watches. If you are sensitive to nickel, chances are you've had a reaction like this at some point in your life.

What you may not know is that nickel allergies can also react internally. The food you eat, how it is stored, what it's cooked in — all of these can lead to an internal reaction to nickel. The symptoms are less noticeable. You may experience a runny nose, headaches, sores or torn skin in the mouth, pain in the stomach or digestive tract, swelling or itching tongue and throat, or a lowered immune system, causing you to get sick regularly.

Both are reactions to nickel, and both can be prevented.

The challenge is to identify items that contain nickel so you can avoid them. External reactions are easier — buy jewelry that states it's nickel free, coat pant buttons and belt buckles with clear nail polish or material, switch to plastic watch bands. If you're not in contact with nickel, you won't react.

Internal reactions are trickier — foods possess a range of nickel levels, certain pans and containers leach nickel into food, mixing some foods together will increase the amount of nickel, your tolerance may be low or high, and exposure to nickel over time can change your tolerance. The best way to prevent an internal reaction is by being mindful of what's going into your body.

This cookbook is meant to help ease the burden of regulating nickel allergies. Included are a list of nickel foods and their corresponding levels to give you a better idea of what to eat and what to avoid, recipes that combine foods together in a safer way, and substitutions and tips to use when you can't find a product that's low-nickel.

This book is specific to nickel allergies, but the recipes can be safely consumed by anyone with an allergy or restriction to foods on the avoid list, including gluten, nut, and soy allergies.

The List

If you want to know what foods you should and should not eat, the following is a list of good foods, foods to eat in moderation, and foods to avoid. It has been compiled from research the FDA conducted on nickel levels in foods, cross-compared to the list of foods from an allergist, and edited with a lot of trial and error.

Keep in mind, though, that many things can affect the nickel level in foods:

- the level of nickel in the ground where the food is grown
- how the food is stored
- how the food is prepared
- what foods you mix together.

The best way to avoid a reaction is to consume and be exposed to less nickel. The following DOs and DON'Ts list will help you find ways to limit your contact with nickel.

DO	DON'T
* Read all labels when food shopping * Check for changes a company may have made to their product * Check medicines and supplements for high nickel foods in their inactive ingredient list * Switch to lower nickel products you use on a regular basis * Use pans made from aluminum, ceramic, glass, magnetic stainless steel, or have a non-stick surface * Try a new food not on the list in a small amount by itself when you've been eating low nickel foods	* Eat food stored in a can * Make food in a stainless steel pan that is not magnetic * Combine moderate nickel foods with a lot of high acid foods, like tomatoes or apples * Mix together too many ingredients * Eat or combine too many moderation foods together * Eat foods high in nickel * Try a new food not on the list when you've been eating moderation nickel foods, combined with other foods, or in large amounts

With nickel allergies, remember the motto: Everything in moderation. The more you eat, the more nickel you consume.

The List

Good	Moderation	Avoid
<u>Dairy</u>	<u>Dairy</u>	<u>Dairy</u>
▸ Butter, salted and unsalted ▸ Cheddar cheese ▸ Cottage cheese ▸ Cream cheese ▸ Cream substitute, non-dairy liquid/frozen ▸ Half and half cream ▸ Heavy whipping cream ▸ Ice cream, French vanilla ▸ Ice cream, New York vanilla ▸ Ice cream, regular vanilla ▸ Milk—whole, low fat, skim ▸ Other cheeses ▸ Sour cream, plain ▸ Swiss cheese ▸ Yogurt (no citric acid or raspberry)	▸ American processed cheese	▸ Chocolate milk ▸ Margarine ▸ Milkshake, chocolate ▸ Sour cream dip

The List

Good	Moderation	Avoid
Fruits	**Fruits**	**Fruits**
▶ Apple juice (no citric acid) ▶ Apple pie (fresh/frozen with rice flour crust) ▶ Apples* ▶ Berries (except raspberries) ▶ Cherries ▶ Cranberries ▶ Cranberry juice cocktail (no citric acid) ▶ Fruit drink (10% juice, no citric acid) ▶ Fruit drink, from powder (no citric acid) ▶ Fruit juice blend (100% juice, no citric acid) ▶ Grape juice (no citric acid) ▶ Grapes ▶ Kiwi ▶ Pears ▶ Rhubarb ▶ Sparkling apple juice (no citric acid) ▶ Sparkling grape juice (no citric acid) ▶ Strawberries	▶ Bananas ▶ Watermelon	▶ Apricots, canned and fresh ▶ Canned pears ▶ Cantaloupe ▶ Dates ▶ Figs ▶ Fruit cocktail, canned and fresh ▶ Grapefruit ▶ Grapefruit juice ▶ Lemonade ▶ Lemons ▶ Limes ▶ Nectarines ▶ Orange juice ▶ Oranges ▶ Peaches ▶ Pineapple juice ▶ Pineapples ▶ Prune juice ▶ Prunes ▶ Raisins ▶ Raspberries ▶ Tangerines

The List

Good	Moderation	Avoid
Vegetables	Vegetables	Vegetables
▶ Brussels sprouts ▶ Cabbage ▶ Celery ▶ Coleslaw, mayonnaise-type (no soy or carrots) ▶ Corn, fresh/frozen or boiled ▶ Cucumbers ▶ Dill cucumber pickles (no garlic) ▶ Eggplant ▶ Green onions ▶ Mushrooms ▶ Okra ▶ Onions ▶ Potatoes, boiled without peel ▶ Potatoes, mashed, prepared from fresh ▶ Potato salad, mayonnaise-type (no soy) ▶ Sweet cucumber pickles ▶ Summer squash, raw and boiled ▶ Tomatoes, raw ▶ Turnips	▶ Beets ▶ Collard greens ▶ Corn, canned ▶ Potatoes, baked without peel ▶ Uncooked pureed tomatoes	▶ Asparagus ▶ Avocados ▶ Baby carrots ▶ Bean sprouts ▶ Black olives ▶ Broccoli ▶ Canned tomato soup ▶ Carrots, fresh, peeled, or boiled ▶ Cauliflower ▶ Garlic ▶ Green beans ▶ Kale ▶ Leafy greens ▶ Leeks ▶ Lettuce ▶ Mixed vegetables ▶ Peas ▶ Peppers, raw or cooked ▶ Potatoes, baked or boiled with peel ▶ Potatoes, French-fried ▶ Pumpkins ▶ Pumpkin pie ▶ Spaghetti sauce ▶ Spinach ▶ Sprouts made from beans or alfalfa ▶ Squash, winter (Hubbard, acorn) ▶ Sweet potatoes ▶ Tomato salsa ▶ Tomato sauce, plain

The List

Good	Moderation	Avoid
Meats	Meats	Meats
▸ Beef roast—chuck, oven-roasted ▸ Beef steak, loin/sirloin ▸ Bologna (beef/pork/chicken) ▸ Chicken breast, oven-roasted (skin removed) ▸ Chicken thigh, oven-roasted (skin removed) ▸ Eggs ▸ Frankfurter (beef/pork), boiled ▸ Ham—cured (not canned), baked ▸ Homemade lasagna, corn noodles with chopped meat ▸ Liver (beef/calf), pan-cooked ▸ Luncheon meat (chicken/turkey) ▸ Luncheon meat (ham) ▸ Pork roast, loin, oven-roasted	▸ Chicken breast, fried with skin ▸ Chicken fillet (broiled), no bun ▸ Chicken pot pie, frozen, heated (rice flour crust) ▸ Lamb chops, pan-cooked with oil ▸ Pork chop, pan-cooked with oil ▸ Pork sausage (link/patty), oven-cooked ▸ Salami, luncheon-meat type (not hard, no garlic) ▸ Turkey breast, oven-roasted	▸ Almonds ▸ Beef and veggie stew, canned ▸ Beef, bean, & cheese burrito ▸ Beef—ground, regular, pan-cooked ▸ Beef stroganoff with noodles ▸ Beef with vegetables in sauce (Chinese take-out) ▸ Boiled or fresh shrimp ▸ Canned chicken noodle soup ▸ Canned tuna ▸ Chicken nuggets, fast-food ▸ Chili con carne with beans ▸ Fish, especially salmon and catfish ▸ Fish sandwich, fast-food ▸ Fish sticks or patty, frozen, oven-cooked ▸ Frozen lasagna, heated ▸ Hazel nuts and other nuts ▸ Lentils ▸ Lima beans ▸ Meatloaf, beef, homemade ▸ New England clam chowder ▸ Peanut butter ▸ Peanuts ▸ Pinto beans ▸ Pork and beans ▸ Quarter pounder cheeseburger on bun ▸ Quarter pounder hamburger on bun ▸ Refried beans ▸ Sesame seeds ▸ Shellfish ▸ Soy protein powder (used in sausages, sandwich meat, minced meat, bread, soup, concentrates, bouillon, etc.) ▸ Soybeans ▸ Sunflower seeds ▸ Taco/tostada with beef and cheese ▸ Tuna noodle casserole ▸ White beans

The List

Good	Moderation	Avoid
Grains	Grains	Grains
▶ Breakfast foods made of white rice or corn (with olive, corn, or canola oil, no soy or citric acid)* ▶ Corn/hominy grits, enriched, cooked ▶ Corn square cereal ▶ Corn tortillas, white and yellow ▶ Cornmeal, white or yellow ▶ Macaroni and cheese, from corn or white rice ▶ Macaroni noodles (corn or white rice) ▶ Noodles, egg from corn or white rice, boiled ▶ Popcorn, air-popped ▶ Rice square cereal ▶ Spaghetti, corn or white rice, boiled ▶ Tortilla chips made from olive, canola, or corn oil	▶ Macaroni salad, from grocery/deli (made with corn or white rice, no soy)* ▶ Muffin, fruit or plain (white rice or corn flour) ▶ Pizza, homemade with white rice flour, no tomato sauce ▶ Rice, white, enriched, cooked	▶ Bagel, plain, toasted ▶ Biscuits ▶ Bran ▶ Bread, cracked wheat ▶ Bread, rye ▶ Bread, white, enriched ▶ Bread, whole wheat ▶ Breakfast tart/toaster pastry ▶ Buckwheat ▶ Butter-type crackers ▶ Corn/tortilla chips ▶ Cornbread, homemade with flour ▶ Cornflakes, cereal ▶ Cream of wheat (farina) ▶ Crisped rice cereal ▶ English muffin, plain, toasted ▶ Fiber products, including cereals, bran biscuits, and fiber tablets ▶ Fried rice, meatless (Chinese take-out) ▶ Frozen, heated pancakes ▶ Fruit-flavored cereal ▶ Graham crackers ▶ Granola bar with raisins ▶ Granola cereal with raisins ▶ Millet ▶ Muesli and other similar breakfast cereals ▶ Multigrain bread ▶ Oat ring cereal (Cheerios) ▶ Oatmeal ▶ Pizza, take-out ▶ Popcorn, microwaved ▶ Pretzels, hard, salted ▶ Raisin bran cereal ▶ Ramen noodles ▶ Rye bread ▶ Saltine crackers ▶ Shredded wheat cereal ▶ Sweet roll/Danish pastry ▶ Tortilla, flour ▶ Unpolished/brown rice ▶ Wheat bran and other bran ▶ Whole grain breads/biscuits

The List

Good	Moderation	Avoid
Other	Other	Other
▸ Beer ▸ Bottled drinking water* ▸ Brown sugar ▸ Candy, hard, any flavor (no raspberry, citric acid, or soy)* ▸ Canola oil ▸ Carbonated beverages (no citric acid) ▸ Coffee, from ground ▸ Corn oil ▸ Cornstarch ▸ Decaf coffee, from ground ▸ Decaf tea, from tea bag (no raspberry or citric acid)* ▸ Dill ▸ Gelatin dessert (Jello, no citric acid or raspberry) ▸ Honey ▸ Italian salad dressing, no soy ▸ Jelly (except raspberry or citric acid) ▸ Mayonnaise (non-soybean type) ▸ Olive oil ▸ Popsicle, fruit flavored* ▸ Potato chips, olive, canola, or corn oil, no garlic or citric acid ▸ Powdered sugar ▸ Rum flavor ▸ Sherbert* ▸ Sugar, white, granulated ▸ Syrup, caramel (no soy) ▸ Tea, from tea bag* ▸ Vanilla ▸ Wine Yeast	▸ Meal replacement drinks (except chocolate)* ▸ Salad dressing, no soy, creamy/buttermilk type* ▸ Syrup, pancake* ▸ Tomato catsup/ ketchup* ▸ Yellow mustard	▸ Baking powder ▸ Brownies ▸ Cake, chocolate with icing ▸ Candy bar, milk chocolate or dark ▸ Candy bar, nougat or nut ▸ Canned/bottled brown gravy ▸ Chocolate and cocoa drinks ▸ Coconut oils ▸ Donuts, flour-type ▸ Linseed and linseed oil ▸ Nut oils ▸ Parsley ▸ Potato chips ▸ Pudding (chocolate or other) ▸ Sandwich cookies with creme filling (Oreos) ▸ Sugar cookies, including gluten free ▸ Sweet and sour sauce ▸ Sweets with chocolate, marzipan, nuts, or strong licorice ▸ Syrup, butterscotch ▸ Syrup, chocolate ▸ Tea from drink dispensers ▸ Vegetable oil ▸ Vitamins with nickel or soy ▸ Yellow cake with icing

*Watch out for hidden ingredients, such as soy, citric acid, raspberry, pineapple, etc.

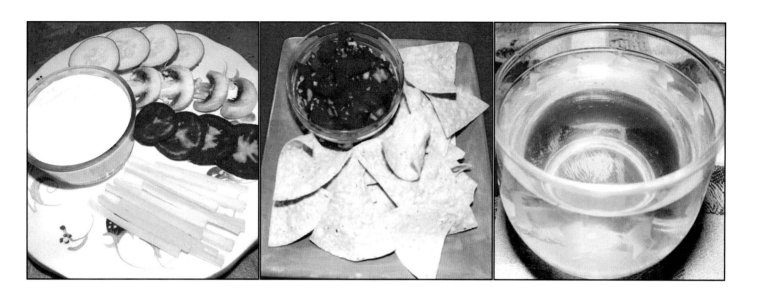

Appetizers, Sides, and Beverages

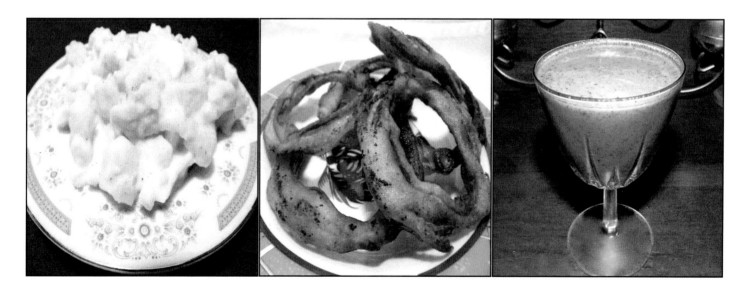

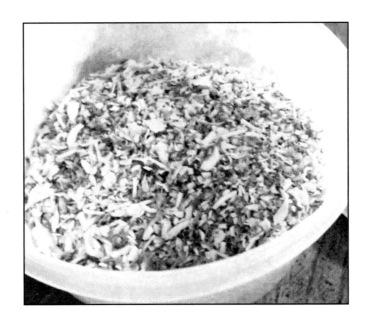

Onion Ranch Dressing Mix

Prep Time: 5 min.

Makes: 2 1/2 cups of mix

1 Tbsp black pepper

1/2 c dried chives

2 Tbsp onion powder

1 c dried minced onions

2 Tbsp dill weed

1 Tbsp celery salt

1. Mix together black pepper, chives, onion powder, minced onions, dill weed, and celery salt.

2. Store in airtight container until ready to make dressing or use as a seasoning.

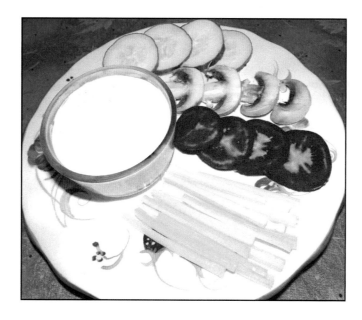

Onion Ranch Dressing

Prep Time: 5 min.

Chill Time: 2 hrs.

Makes: 1 3/4 quarts

1 c mayonnaise

1 c buttermilk

3/4 c sour cream

1 1/2 Tbsp dry ranch dressing mix (p.2)

1. Mix together mayonnaise, buttermilk, sour cream, and dry ranch dressing mix until smooth.

2. Chill 2 hrs. before use. Store in the refrigerator.

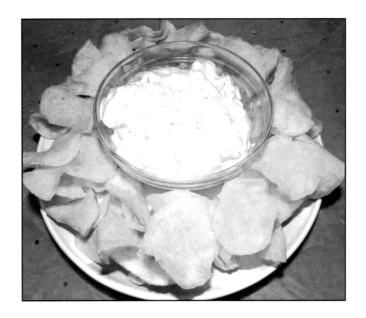

Cool Cucumber Dip

Prep Time: 5 min.

Makes: I cup

I c sour cream

1/4 c mayonnaise

1/2 medium cucumber, peeled, seeded, and chopped

I Tbsp fresh minced dill OR 1/4 tsp dill weed

sprinkle of salt and pepper

1. In a medium bowl, combine sour cream and mayonnaise.

2. Add cucumber and dill, stirring until smooth. Season with salt and pepper. Serve cold.

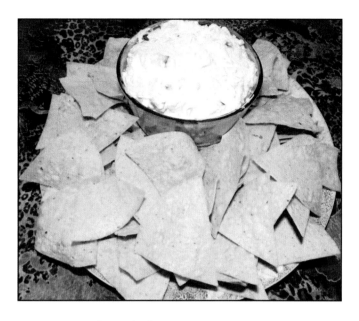

Cool Gazpacho Dip

Prep Time: 5 min.

Chill Time: 2-3 hrs.

Makes: 12 servings

1 pkg (8 oz) cream cheese, softened

1/4 c sour cream

1/2 c shredded cheddar cheese

2 Tbsp minced fresh cilantro

1 small tomato, seeded and chopped

2 green onions, sliced

1/3 c cucumber, chopped

1. In medium bowl, mix cream cheese and sour cream together. Stir in cheddar cheese and cilantro. Cover and chill 2-3 hours.

2. Place in serving dish. Top with tomato, onions, and cucumber. Serve with tortilla chips.

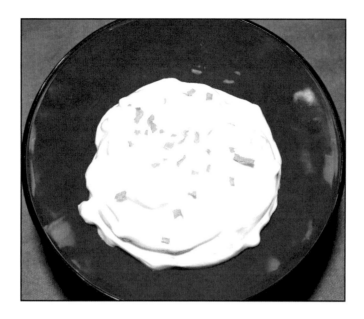

French Onion Dip

Prep Time: 5 min.

Makes: 1 cup

1 c sour cream

1 tsp seasoning salt

1-2 Tbsp dry onion flakes

1. Blend together sour cream and seasoning salt. Stir in onion flakes until completely blended.

2. Chill until ready to use. Use on chips or with fresh veggie slices.

Variations: Can use 1 green onion sprig in place of dry onion flakes.

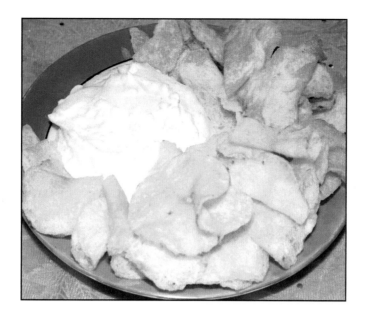

Sweet Green Onion Dip

Prep Time: 5 min.

Makes: 1 cup

1 c sour cream

1/4 c diced green onion sprig

1 tsp sugar

1 tsp seasoning salt

1 tsp onion powder

1. Combine sour cream and diced green onion in a bowl. Add sugar, seasoning salt, and onion powder; mix.

2. Serve chilled with either tortilla chips or potato chips.

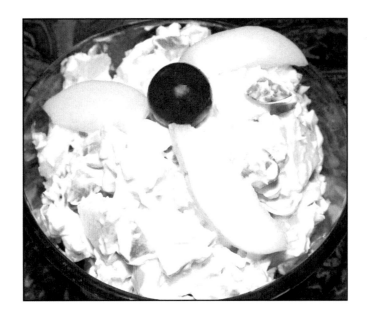

Apple Dip

Prep Time: 5 min.

Makes: 2 cups

I Tbsp packed brown sugar

I pkg (8 oz) cream cheese, softened

I medium apple, cored and chopped

I medium pear, cored and chopped

1/2 c chopped seedless red grapes

1/4 c chopped celery

1. Blend together brown sugar and cream cheese in a medium bowl. Stir in apple, pear,

grapes, and celery.

2. Chill and serve. Best used as a dip for cinnamon chips.

Variations: Can use white sugar in place of brown sugar.

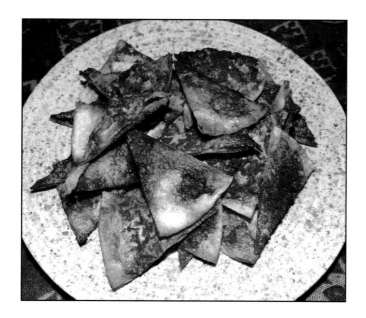

Cinnamon Chips

Prep Time: 5 min.
Cook Time: 5-7 min.
Makes: 32 chips

2 Tbsp sugar

1/2 tsp ground cinnamon

4 (8-in) white or yellow corn tortillas

1. Preheat oven to 425°F. Mix sugar and cinnamon in small bowl.

2. Wet tortillas lightly with water. Sprinkle sugar mixture evenly on each tortilla and rub in.

3. Cut into 8 even pieces. Grease baking sheet and arrange, not overlapping. Bake 5-7 min. until golden brown, watching carefully the last 2 min. to keep from burning. Cool completely before eating.

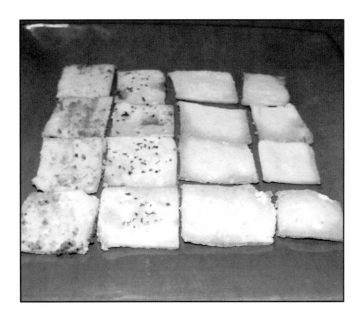

Soda Crackers

Prep Time: 20 min.
Cook Time: 10 min.
Makes: about 56 crackers

2 c all-purpose rice flour blend

1 tsp salt

1/2 tsp baking soda

1/4 c butter

1/2 c sour milk

1 tsp vinegar

1 large egg

1. Preheat oven to 400°F. Sift together rice flour, salt, and baking soda. Cut in butter until crumbly. Add sour milk, vinegar, and egg. Stir until it makes a dough.

2. On floured surface, roll out dough thin. Cut into squares and place on greased baking pan. Bake for 10 min. or until browned.

Variations: Salted crackers—add salt to top. Chicken crackers—combine 1 tsp chicken base, 1 tsp onion powder, and 1 tsp cilantro. Add to top. Cheese crackers—melt 2 Tbsp butter, mix with 1/4 c parmesan cheese. Brush on top.

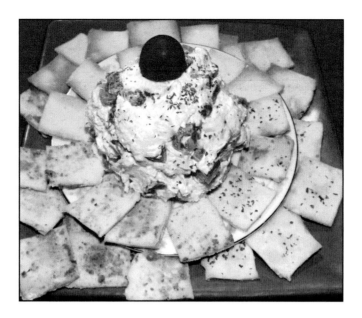

Holiday Cheese Ball

Prep Time: 15 min.

Chill Time: 1 hr.

Makes: 1 large cheese ball

2 c cream cheese, softened

2 c sharp cheddar cheese, shredded

1/4 c Colby cheese, shredded

3 Tbsp finely chopped onions

3 Tbsp tomato, seeded and chopped

1 tsp onion powder

1. Beat cream cheese in medium bowl. Add cheddar cheese, Colby cheese, onions, tomato, and onion powder. Mix until blended.

2. Cover bowl and refrigerate 1 hr. Shape into one big ball or several smaller balls. Keep chilled.

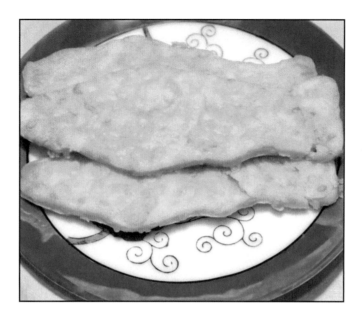

Goldfish Crackers

Prep Time: 30 min.

Cook Time: 15 min.

Makes: 7 dozen crackers

2 c cheddar cheese, shredded

4 Tbsp butter, cubed

1 c all-purpose rice flour blend

3/4 tsp salt

3 Tbsp cold water

1. Preheat oven to 350°F. Mix together cheese, butter, rice flour, and salt until crumbly. Mix in water, a little at a time.

2. Chill in refrigerator for 20 min. Roll out dough on floured surface. Cut into desired shapes.

3. Place on greased baking sheet. Cook 15 min. until crispy.

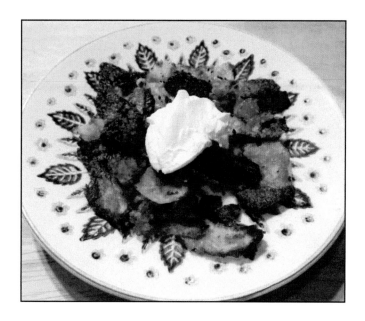

Potato Crisps

Prep Time: 10 min.

Cook Time: 15-20 min.

Makes: 24-30 pieces

4 medium baking potatoes, peeled

1 Tbsp canola or olive oil

sprinkle salt or seasoning salt

sour cream for dipping (optional)

1. Preheat oven to 400°F. Cut potatoes into 1/4-in. thick slices.

2. In a large bowl, add oil to potatoes; mix. Add salt, coat evenly. Arrange potato slices on greased baking sheet, not overlapping.

3. Bake 15-20 min. or until soft. Serve warm with sour cream if desired.

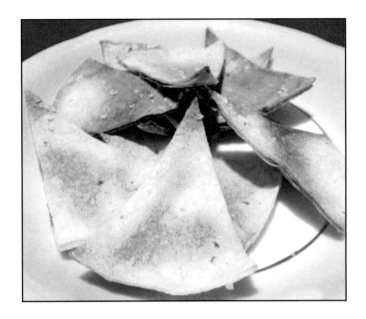

Baked Tortilla Chips

Prep Time: 5 min.

Cook Time: 5-7 min.

Makes: 56 chips

7 (8-in) white or yellow corn tortillas

salt to taste

1. Preheat oven to 425°F. Wet tortillas lightly with water. Sprinkle salt to taste.

2. Cut into 8 triangular pieces each. Arrange on greased baking sheet so they don't overlap.

3. Bake 5-7 min. until crispy, watching carefully the last 2 min. to keep from burning. Remove and cool.

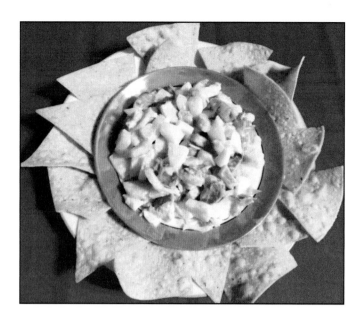

Creamy Cucumber Salsa

Prep Time: 15 min.

Makes: 3 cups

2 cucumbers, peeled, seeded, and chopped

2 tomatoes, seeded and finely chopped

1 small onion, finely chopped

1/4 c celery leaves, chopped fine

1/4 c sour cream

1/2 tsp seasoning salt

1 tsp onion powder

1 tsp white vinegar

2 Tbsp mayonnaise

1 tsp sugar

1/2 tsp celery salt

1/2 tsp salt

1. In bowl, combine cucumber, tomatoes, onions, and celery leaves. Set aside.

2. In small bowl, combine sour cream, seasoning salt, onion powder, vinegar, mayonnaise, sugar, celery salt, and salt. Pour over vegetables and coat. Serve fresh.

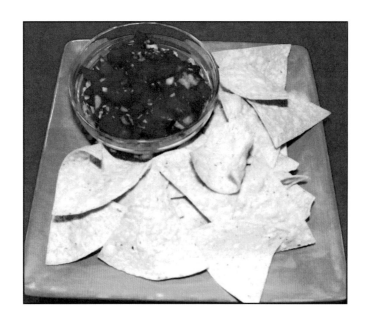

Fresh Salsa
Prep Time: 5 min.
Makes: 1 cup

2 Tbsp ketchup

1 Tbsp balsamic vinegar

1 tomato, diced

1 sprig green onion, diced

1 tsp onion powder

1 tsp onion flakes

1. In small bowl, combine ketchup and balsamic vinegar. Stir in tomatoes and green onions until coated.

2. Add onion powder and onion flakes, stirring until incorporated. Serve chilled.

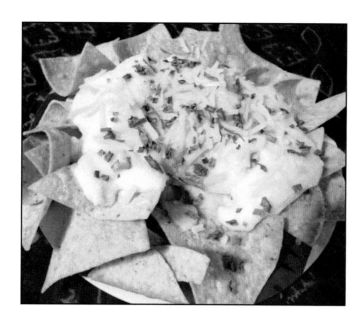

Nachos

Prep Time: 5 min.
Cook Time: 5-10 min.
Makes: 2 cups

2 Tbsp butter

1 Tbsp all-purpose rice flour blend

1 c milk

1 c cheddar cheese, shredded

tortilla chips

1/2 c sour cream (optional)

chopped chives to taste (optional)

1. Melt butter in saucepan. Whisk in rice flour. Cook until slightly browned. Whisk in milk, 1/2 c at a time. Add cheese.

2. Cook until cheese is melted, stirring constantly. Serve hot over tortilla chips. Can top with sour cream and chives if desired.

Variations: Can use white or yellow corn meal in place of all-purpose rice flour blend.

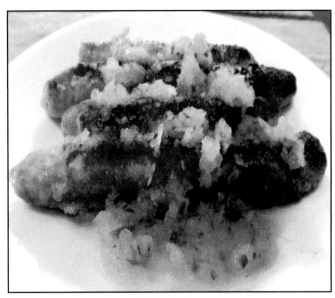

Relish

Prep Time: 20 min.

Chill Time: 8 hrs.

Makes: 5 pints

5 c cucumber, ground

3 c onions, ground

3 c celery, ground

2 Tbsp celery salt

2 c water

1 quart white vinegar

3 c sugar

2 tsp mustard seed

1. Combine cucumber, onions, and celery in container. Add celery salt and water. Let stand overnight for about 8 hrs in refrigerator; drain.

2. In large saucepan, heat vinegar, sugar, and mustard seed to boiling. Stir in vegetable mix, bringing to a boil. Cook slowly 10 min. Can keep in the refrigerator or store in canning jars.

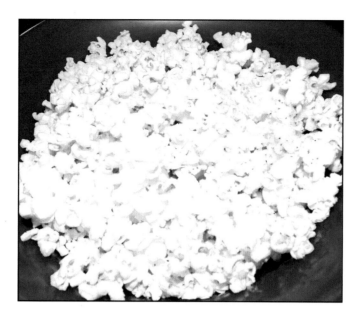

Loaded Popcorn

Prep Time: 5 min.

Cook Time: 5 min.

Makes: 1 serving bowl of popcorn

1/2 c unpopped popcorn

2 Tbsp melted butter

1 tsp salt

1 tsp seasoning salt

1 tsp pepper

1 Tbsp sugar

1. In air popper, pop the popcorn into a large bowl. Coat with melted butter.

2. Sprinkle on salt, seasoning salt, pepper, and sugar. Toss until mixed. Serve warm.

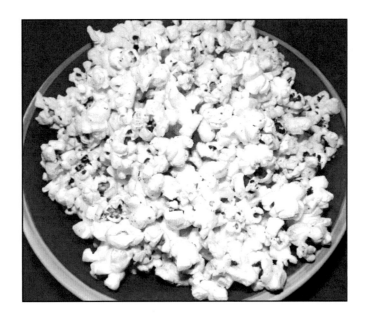

Bacon Kettle Popcorn

Prep Time: 5 min.

Cook Time: 5-10 min.

Makes: 1 serving bowl of popcorn

bacon drippings* (enough for bottom of kettle)

1/2 c unpopped popcorn

1 tsp sugar

1 tsp salt

1/4 c melted butter

*Add some extra canola oil to drippings if not enough

1. Heat the grease in a covered kettle. Add popcorn before it's too hot. Cover and wait for it to start popping.

2. Shake kettle's handle to keep it from sticking. Once popped, remove from heat and put into a serving bowl.

3. Add sugar, salt, and melted butter to the top. Serve warm.

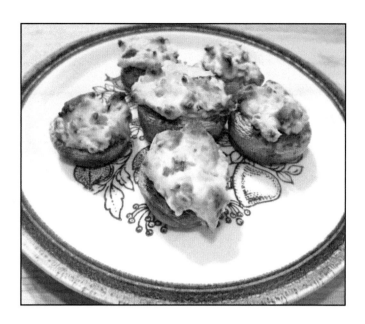

Stuffed Mushrooms

Prep Time: 10 min.

Cook Time: 18-20 min.

Makes: 24-30 stuffed mushrooms

2 lbs medium or large fresh mushrooms

1 pkg (8 oz) cream cheese, softened

1/2 c cheddar cheese, shredded

1/2 c cooked ham, chopped

1. Preheat oven to 400°F. Pull off stems of mushrooms. Place caps stem-side up on greased baking sheet. Chop mushroom stems to make 1/2 c.

2. In medium bowl, cream together cream cheese and cheddar cheese. Add chopped mushroom stems and ham; mix. Spoon into mushroom caps, gently pressing it in.

3. Bake 18-20 min. or until golden brown.

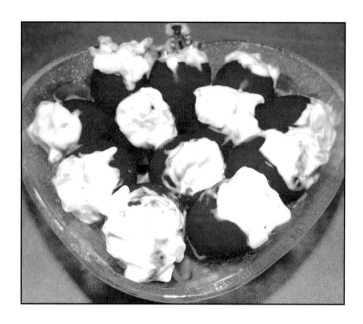

Stuffed Cherry Tomatoes

Prep Time: 15 min.

Chill Time: 2 hrs.

Makes: 24 stuffed cherry tomatoes

24 cherry tomatoes, no stems

6 bacon slices, cooked, drained, & crumbled

1/2 c finely chopped green onions

1/2 c mayonnaise

1. Slice off the tops of each tomato. Scoop out tomato seeds. Let tomatoes drain on a paper towel.

2. In small bowl, mix bacon, onions, and mayonnaise together. Spoon into each tomato.

3. Cover and chill for 2 hrs. Serve cold.

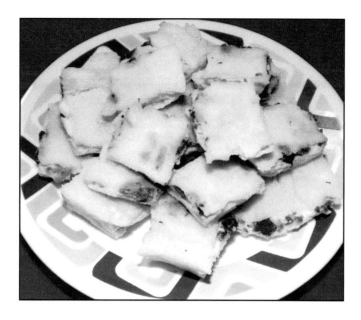

Creamy Bacon Bites

Prep Time: 15 min.

Cook Time: 20 min.

Makes: 32 bites

1 ball all-purpose rice flour dough (p.182)

1 pkg (8 oz) cream cheese, softened

4 slices bacon, cooked, drained, and crumbled

2 Tbsp chopped onions

sprinkle black pepper

1. Preheat oven to 350°F. Roll dough on floured surface, about 1/4-in. thick. Set aside.

2. In small bowl, combine cream cheese, bacon, onions, and black pepper. Carefully spread onto dough. Fold dough over, pressing the seams together. Slice and roll into 1-in. pieces.

3. Brush on melted butter. Place on greased baking sheet. Bake 15 min., turn over, and bake 5 more min. or until golden on both sides. Serve warm.

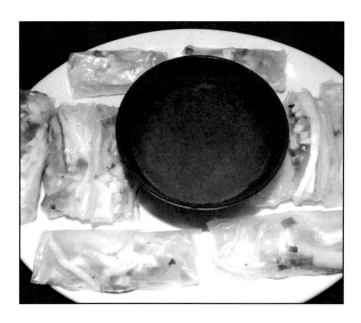

Cabbage Spring Rolls

Prep Time: 20 min.
Chill Time: 30 min.
Makes: 20-30 rolls

warm water
1 pkg rice paper
2 c cabbage, julienned
1 c green onion, chopped
1 c celery, julienned
1 c onions, julienned
1 c mushrooms, diced
1 c cucumber, julienned
dipping sauce (p.25)

1. In jellyroll pan, pour in warm water. Dip rice paper in for 2 seconds and place on a cutting board for wrapping.

2. On the top of the wrap, place down some cabbage. Layer on green onions, celery, onions, mushroom, and cucumber. Don't overfill. Wrap, starting at the top, tucking under the ingredients, fold in the sides, and roll. Repeat for each roll. Place on plate and chill 30 min. Eat with sauce.

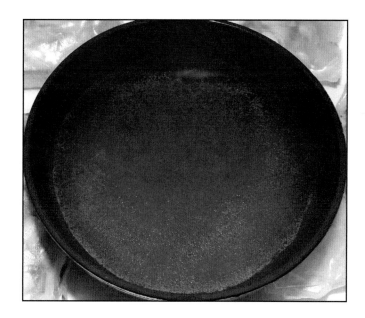

Dipping Sauce

Prep Time: 5 min.

Cook Time: 10 min.

Makes: 1 cup

1/2 c white wine vinegar

1 tsp mirin or rice vinegar

1 Tbsp brown sugar

2 tsp cornstarch dissolved in 1/2 c cold water

1/2 tsp salt

1 Tbsp white sugar

1. In saucepan, combine white wine vinegar, mirin, brown sugar, cornstarch mixture, salt, and white sugar.

2. Cook on medium heat until sauce becomes brown and smooth, about 10 min. Serve with cabbage spring rolls (see recipe).

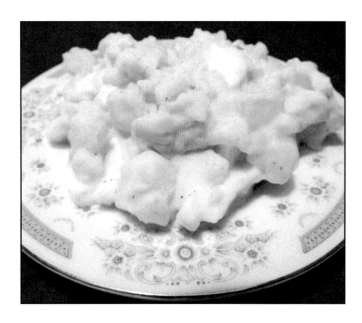

Deviled Egg Potato Salad

Prep Time: 20 min.

Makes: 3-4 servings

2 c potatoes, peeled, sliced, and boiled

1/4 c onions, diced

1/2 c mayonnaise or salad dressing

1 Tbsp sugar

1/2 tsp salt

1/4 tsp pepper

1 tsp yellow mustard

2 eggs, boiled and peeled

1. In bowl, combine potatoes, onions, mayonnaise, sugar, salt, and pepper. Stir until coated.

2. Add mustard; stir. Slice eggs with egg slicer and add to bowl; stir until incorporated. Serve chilled.

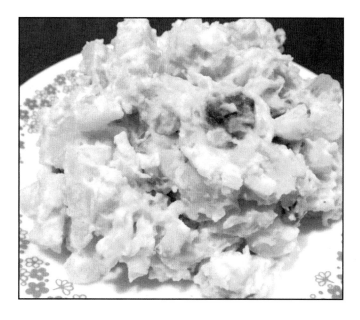

Loaded Baked Potato Salad

Prep Time: 25 min.

Makes: 4 servings

1/4 c sour cream

1/4 c mayonnaise

green or red onions, to taste

1/3 c cheddar cheese, shredded

2 1/2 c potatoes, peeled, sliced, and boiled

1/2 c bacon, cooked and crumbled

1/4 tsp salt

1/4 c yellow onions, chopped

1. In bowl, combine sour cream, mayonnaise, green onions, and cheese.

2. Add potatoes, bacon, salt, and yellow onions. Stir until potatoes are completely coated.

Serve cold.

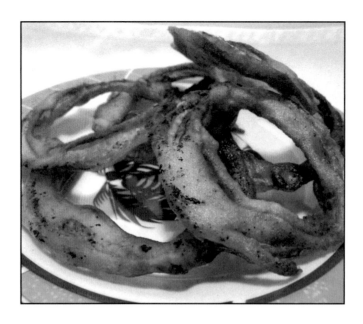

Fried Onion Rings

Prep Time: 15 min.
Cook Time: 30 min.
Makes: 3-4 dozen rings

1 c all-purpose rice flour blend
1/4 tsp baking soda
2 Tbsp sugar
1/4 tsp salt
1 large egg, beaten
1 c buttermilk
1/2 c milk
1/4 tsp vinegar
1 c canola oil for pan
2 c sliced onion rings

1. In bowl, combine rice flour, baking soda, sugar, and salt. Set aside. In a large bowl, combine egg, buttermilk, milk, and vinegar. Add to flour mixture, stirring until incorporated.

2. In saucepan, heat the oil. When hot, dip each onion ring in batter and place in oil. Cook on both sides until golden brown. Cool slightly.

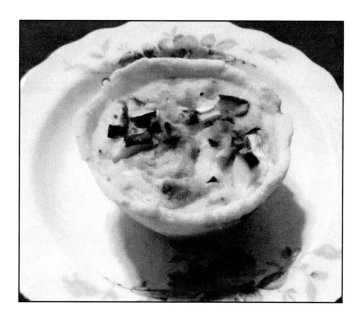

Delicious Mini Quiches

Prep Time: 15 min.
Cook Time: 18-20 min.
Makes: 12 mini quiches

1 ball all-purpose rice flour dough (p.182)

2 eggs

1/2 c milk

1 c chopped zucchini

1/2 c chopped fresh mushrooms

1/2 c shredded cheddar cheese

1/4 c cooked, crumbled bacon

1/4 c sliced green onions

dash black pepper

1. Preheat oven to 375°F. Roll out dough into balls. Press into greased muffin tins.

2. In bowl, whisk eggs and milk. Add zucchini, mushrooms, cheese, bacon, onions, and pepper, stirring together.

3. Fill each cup with the mixture. Bake 18-20 min. or until puffy and lightly browned. Cool, remove carefully, and serve warm.

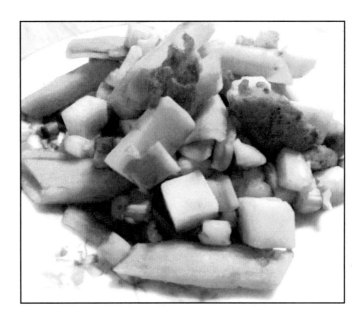

Pasta Chicken Salad

Prep Time: 20 min.

Makes: 4 cups

2 c cooked corn penne noodles

1 c fried chicken, cubed (p.82)

1 c mozzarella cheese, cubed

1/2 c green onions, chopped

1 Tbsp blueberry balsamic vinegar

2 Tbsp olive oil

1. In bowl, mix penne, chicken cubes, mozzarella cheese, and green onions together. Set aside.

2. In small bowl, mix blueberry balsamic vinegar with olive oil. Pour over noodle mixture and blend until incorporated. Serve chilled.

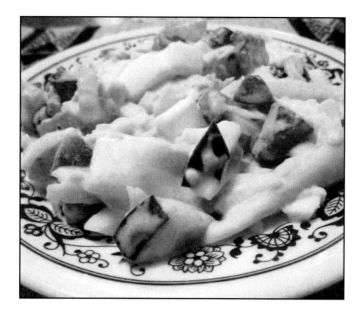

Macaroni/Penne Salad

Prep Time: 10 min.

Cook Time: 10 min.

Makes: 8 cups

1 lb corn elbow noodles/corn penne noodles

1 c pickle juice

1 c boiled eggs, diced

1 c mild cheddar cheese, cubed or shredded

1 c onions, diced

1 c cucumber, diced

1 c sweet pickles, diced OR bread and butters

1 c celery, diced

1 c tomato, diced

1 c mayonnaise

1/2 c milk

salt and pepper to taste

1. Cook noodles until tender. Drain, rinse with cold water. Cool and marinade with pickle juice.

2. Add all other ingredients and stir together. Serve chilled.

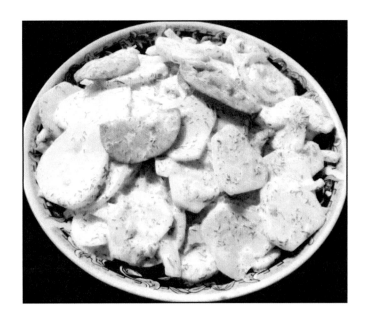

German Cucumber Salad

Prep Time: 10 min.
Chill Time: 2 hrs.
Makes: 6 servings

2 large cucumbers, peeled and thinly sliced

1 small onion, peeled and thinly sliced

4 small Roma tomatoes, thinly sliced

1/3 c sour cream

1/4 tsp mustard

1 Tbsp white vinegar

2 Tbsp milk

3/4 tsp sugar

2 Tbsp dill

salt and pepper to taste

1. In bowl, combine cucumbers, onions, and tomatoes. Set aside.

2. In small bowl, whip together sour cream, mustard, white vinegar, milk, sugar, dill, salt, and pepper.

Pour over vegetables. Toss to coat.

3. Chill 2 hrs. before serving.

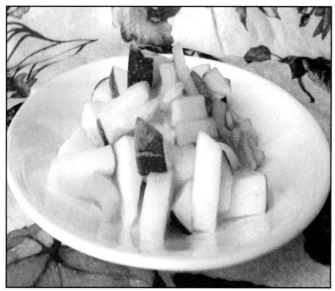

Apple Salad

Prep Time: 15 min.

Cook Time: 10 min.

Makes: 3-4 cups

2 c apples, cored and cubed

1 c celery, sliced

2 Tbsp apple cider vinegar

1 c cold water

1 Tbsp cornstarch

1/4 c white sugar

1. Place apples and celery pieces in water; set aside. In a small saucepan, mix apple cider vinegar, water, cornstarch, and white sugar. Whisk until smooth. Cook on medium heat, stirring constantly until it thickens. Cool for about 10 min.

2. Drain apples and celery. Pour sauce on top and mix. Serve chilled.

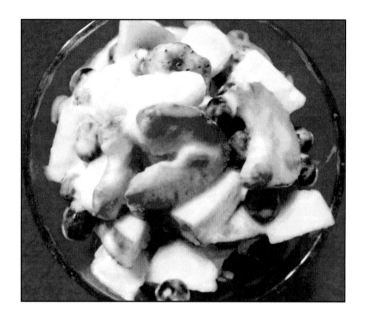

Fruit Salad

Prep Time: 5 min.

Makes: 6 cups

1 c red grapes, sliced in half

1 c apples, chopped

1 c pears, chopped

1 c blueberries

1 c strawberries, sliced

1 c plain yogurt

2-3 Tbsp caramel syrup or sauce (p.169)

1. Mix together grapes, apples, pears, blueberries, strawberries, yogurt, and caramel syrup until incorporated.

2. Serve chilled.

Variations: Use 1/2 c sugar in place of caramel syrup/sauce.

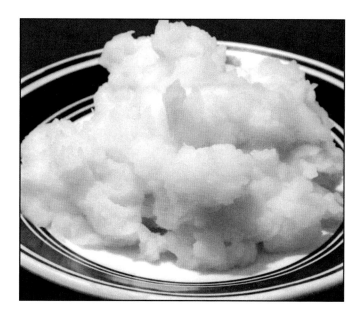

Mashed Potatoes

Prep Time: 10 min.

Cook Time: 20 min.

Makes: 1 serving

1 c peeled and diced potatoes

1/2 Tbsp butter

2 Tbsp milk

dash salt

1. Place potatoes in pot. Fill with water, just covering the potatoes. Place on medium heat and cook until soft.

2. Drain potatoes. Add butter, milk, and salt. Mash with masher or whip with beater until smooth.

Variations: Can add 1 tsp onion powder for a more oniony flavor.

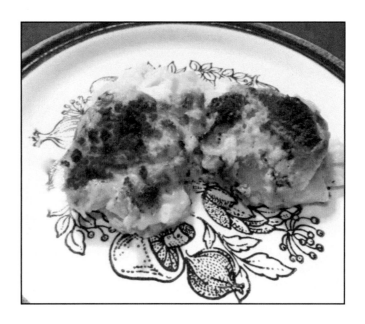

Parmesan Potato au Gratin

Prep Time: 15 min.

Cook Time: 45-50 min.

Makes: 12 servings

2 Tbsp onions, finely chopped

2 c half and half

1 c parmesan cheese

1/2 tsp salt

1/2 tsp pepper

1 Tbsp thyme

2-3 medium potatoes, peeled and thinly sliced

1. Preheat oven to 400°F. Spray muffin tins with cooking spray, set aside. In medium bowl, mix together onions, half and half, 1/2 c parmesan, salt, pepper, and thyme. Set aside.

2. Layer potato slices in muffin tins, keeping it level with the top of the tin. Pour mixture over each potato stack, not overfilling it.

3. Sprinkle remaining parmesan over each stack. Bake 45-50 min. or until cheese is golden brown.

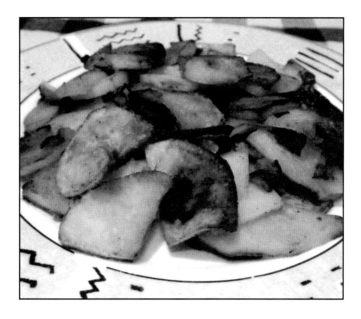

Fried Potato and Onion

Prep Time: 10 min.

Cook Time: 15 min.

Makes: 1 serving

2 Tbsp canola or olive oil

1 c potatoes, peeled and thinly sliced

1/4 c diced or sliced onions

1/2 tsp salt

1/2 tsp pepper

1. Heat oil in skillet. Add potatoes, onions, salt, and pepper.

2. Fry until potatoes are golden and tender. Serve hot.

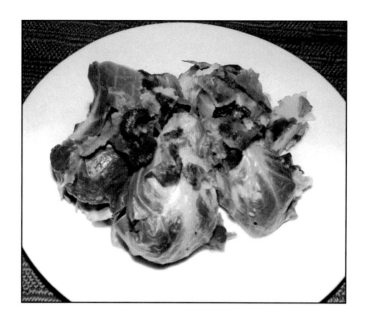

Bacon Brussels Sprouts

Prep Time: 5 min.

Cook Time: 10 min.

Makes: 3-4 servings

1 lb brussels sprouts

2 Tbsp butter

1/2 c bacon, cut into small pieces

1/2 c onions, chopped

1. Boil brussels sprouts in water until tender with fork; drain. In a skillet, fry bacon and onions together until bacon is crisp and onions are golden.

2. Add butter to brussels sprouts and toss until all sprouts are coated. Add bacon and onions to top. Serve hot.

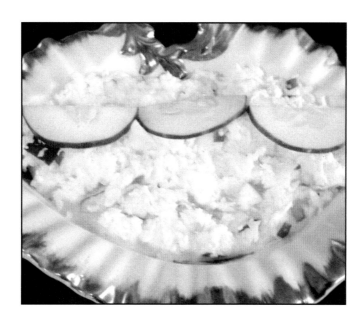

Coleslaw

Prep Time: 20 min.

Chill Time: 1 hr.

Makes: 3 cups

2 c cabbage, shredded

1 onion, sliced thin

1/2 c cucumber, diced

1/2 c mayonnaise

1 tsp sugar

2 Tbsp milk

1/8 tsp salt (optional)

1. In bowl, mix together cabbage, onions, cucumber, and mayonnaise. Add sugar, milk, and salt. Stir until incorporated.

2. Chill for an hour before serving.

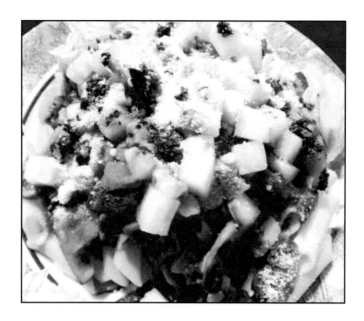

Veggie Delight Pasta

Prep Time: 15 min.
Cook Time: 15 min.
Makes: 4 servings

2 Tbsp olive oil

1 c summer squash, julienned or sliced thin

1 c zucchini, julienned or sliced thin

3/4 c large mushrooms, sliced

1/2 c onions, chopped

1 tsp chicken base

1 tsp Italian seasoning

1 Tbsp balsamic vinegar

2 c corn penne pasta, cooked and drained

parmesan cheese to taste

1/2 c Roma tomatoes, diced (optional)

1. Heat olive oil in a pan. Add squash, zucchini, mushrooms, and onions. Sauté until soft and golden brown. Add chicken base, Italian seasoning, and balsamic vinegar. Cook 1-2 min.

2. Plate penne noodles, top with vegetables. Add parmesan to taste. *Do not cook or reheat tomatoes.

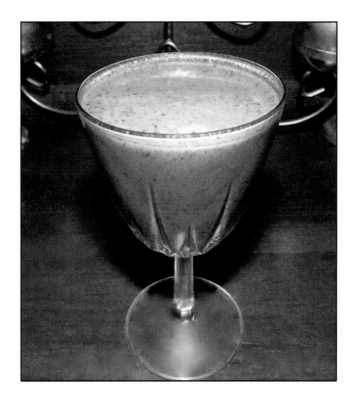

Fruit Shake

Prep Time: 5 min.

Makes: 2 1/2 cups

1 c milk

1 c fresh or frozen strawberries

1 c fresh or frozen blueberries

1/2 c plain yogurt

1 Tbsp sugar

1/2 tsp vanilla extract

4 ice cubes (if using fresh fruit)

1. Blend together milk, strawberries, blueberries, yogurt, sugar, and vanilla.

2. Once smooth, add ice cubes. Blend until thick. Serve chilled.

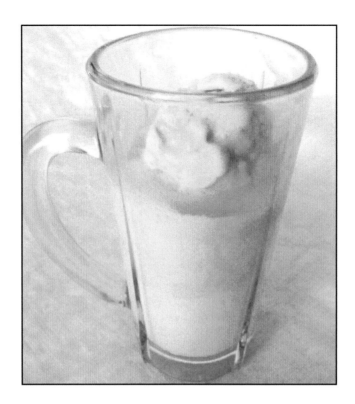

Yogurt Shake

Prep Time: 5 min.

Makes: 4 cups

2 c milk

1 c plain yogurt

1 c vanilla ice cream

2 tsp vanilla extract

1 Tbsp honey

1. Put milk, yogurt, vanilla ice cream, and vanilla extract into blender. Blend until smooth.

2. Add honey. Blend until mixed thoroughly. Serve cold.

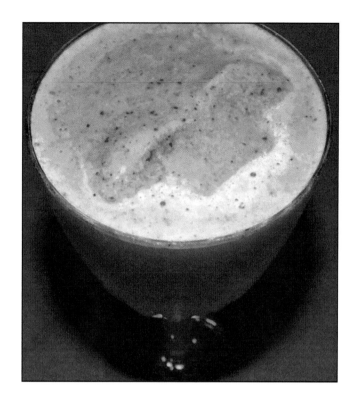

Summer Fruit Smoothie

Prep Time: 5 min.

Makes: 3 cups

1/2 c milk

1/2 c cold apple juice

2 c fresh fruit (strawberries, pears, blueberries)

2 Tbsp sugar

1/2 tsp vanilla extract

10 ice cubes

1. In blender, place milk, apple juice, fresh fruit, sugar, and vanilla extract. Cover and blend until smooth.

2. Add ice cubes. Blend until thick. Serve cold.

Variations: Can use frozen fruit and exclude ice cubes.

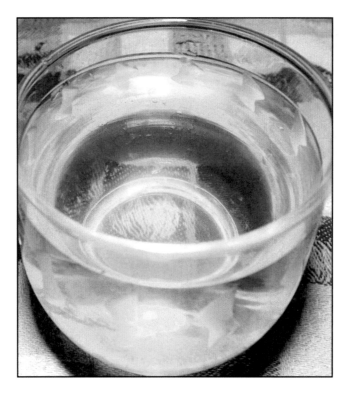

Iced Tea

Prep Time: 10 min.
Chill Time: 2 hrs.
Makes: 8-9 cups

4 c boiling water
2 tea bags (regular, green, or preferred blend)
2 Tbsp honey
4 c cold water
15-20 ice cubes

1. Add boiling water to pitcher. Place tea bags in and steep 5 minutes. Add honey to hot water, stirring until blended.

2. Add cold water and ice. Refrigerate until chilled, about 2 hrs. Serve cold or with ice.

Variations: Can leave out honey for a more robust flavor, or can substitute in 1/2 c sugar for honey.

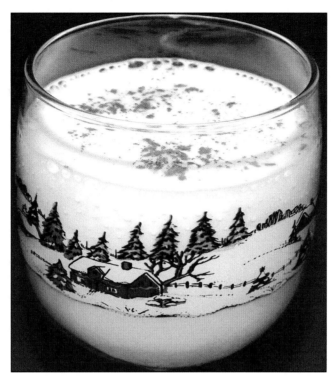

Quick Egg Nog

Prep Time: 5 min.

Chill Time: 1-2 hrs.

Makes: 10 cups

6 c milk

4 eggs, beaten

1 tsp vanilla extract

1 tsp rum extract

1/2 c sugar

1/2 c brandy (optional)

1 tsp cinnamon (optional)

1. In blender, mix milk, eggs, vanilla extract, and rum extract. Blend until smooth. Add sugar and blend.

2. Cover and refrigerate 1-2 hrs. Serve, stirring in brandy and cinnamon, if desired. Pour into glasses.

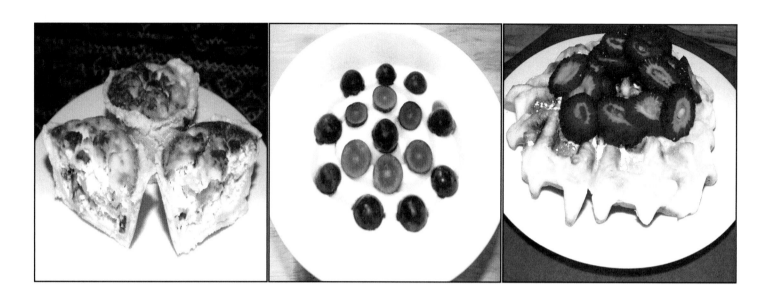

Main Dishes —Breakfast

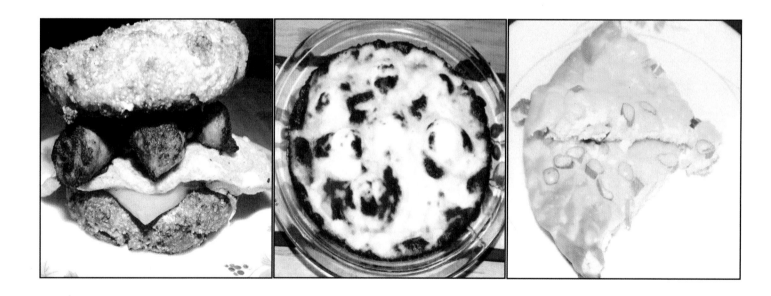

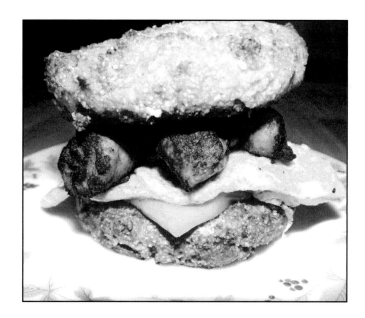

Sausage, Egg, & Cheese Breakfast Biscuit

Prep Time: 15 min.

Cook Time: 10 min.

Makes: 4 servings

5 eggs, beaten

salt and pepper to taste

4 Johnny Cake Biscuits (p.181)

4 slices of cheese

8 sausage links, cooked

1. In bowl, combine eggs, salt, and pepper. Pour mixture in skillet, making 4 equal egg folds. Make sure to cook eggs on both sides.

2. Slice each biscuit in half. Top on one biscuit a slice of cheese, 1 egg fold, and 2 halved sausage links. Top with other biscuit half. Serve warm.

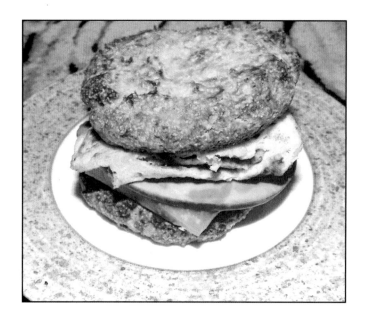

Ham, Egg, & Cheese Breakfast Biscuit

Prep Time: 15 min.

Cook Time: 10 min.

Makes: 4 servings

5 eggs, beaten

salt and pepper to taste

4 Johnny Cake Biscuits (p.181)

4 slices of cheese

4 ham slices

1. In bowl, combine eggs, salt, and pepper. Pour mixture in skillet, making 4 equal egg folds. Make sure to cook eggs on both sides.

2. Slice each biscuit in half. Top on one biscuit a slice of cheese, 1 egg fold, and 1 ham slice. Top with other biscuit half. Serve warm.

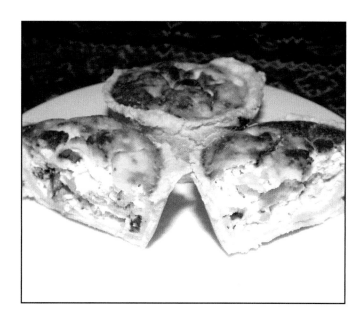

Brunch Tarts

Prep Time: 20 min.
Cook Time: 45 min.
Makes: 4-6 servings

2 Tbsp olive oil

1/2 medium onion, chopped

1/2 c mushrooms, chopped

3 large eggs

1 tsp thyme

salt and pepper to taste

1 (15 oz) container of Ricotta cheese

1 ball pie dough/all-purpose dough (p.182)

1. Preheat oven to 375°F. In large pan, sauté onions and mushrooms in olive oil, about 5 min.

In a bowl, beat 2 eggs, thyme, salt, pepper, and cheese together. Fold in onions and

mushrooms. Mix well.

2. Press dough into greased pie tin or baking pan. Brush remaining beaten egg into crust.

Pour in mixture. Bake 45 min. until golden brown. Let cool 10 minutes before serving.

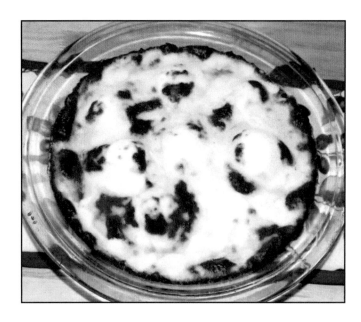

Eggs Mornay

Prep Time: 20 min.

Cook Time: 20-25 min.

Makes: 4-6 servings

8 hard boiled eggs, peeled and halved

1/4 c butter

1/4 c all-purpose rice flour blend

1 1/2 c milk

1/2 c heavy cream

salt and pepper to taste

3/4 c shredded Swiss cheese

1/3 c shredded parmesan cheese

1. Preheat oven to 450°F. Grease a 9-in. baking pan. Place egg slices cut-side down in pan.

2. In saucepan, melt butter. Add rice flour, cook and stir 1 min. Whisk in milk. Cook until boiling, stirring constantly. When thickened, stir in cream, salt, and pepper. Add Swiss cheese, stir until melted.

3. Pour sauce over eggs. Sprinkle with parmesan cheese. Bake 20-25 min. until golden brown.

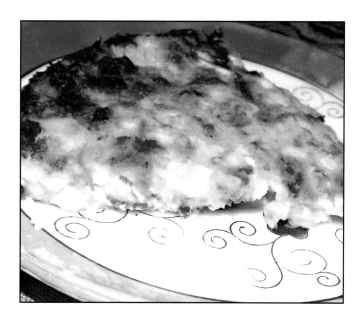

All-in-One Omelet

Prep Time: 20 min.

Cook Time: 35-40 min.

Makes: 4 servings

12 slices bacon, cooked and crumbled

1/2 c onions, chopped

1 c shredded Colby cheese

1/2 c all-purpose rice flour blend

4 eggs

1 1/2 c milk

1/4 tsp salt

dash pepper

1. Preheat oven to 400°F. Grease a pie plate or pan. Sprinkle bacon, onion, and cheese into plate.

2. In bowl, beat together rice flour, eggs, milk, salt, and pepper until smooth. Pour into pie plate or pan. Bake 35-40 min. or until cooked in the middle. Eat warm.

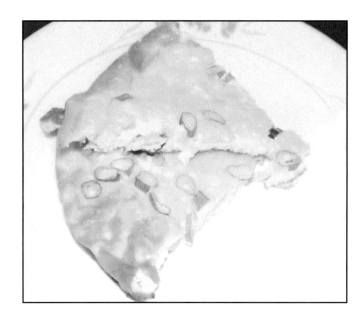

Oven Omelets

Prep Time: 5 min.
Cook Time: 35-40 min.
Makes: 12 servings

1/4 c butter, melted

18 eggs

1 c sour cream

1 c milk

1 1/2 tsp salt or seasoning salt

1/4 c green onions, chopped

1. Preheat oven to 325°F. Use melted butter to coat a 9x13 pan or pie plate. Mix eggs, sour cream, milk, and salt in large bowl.

2. Add green onions, mixing well. Pour mixture into pan or pie plate. Bake 35-40 min. or until the eggs are set. Cut and serve.

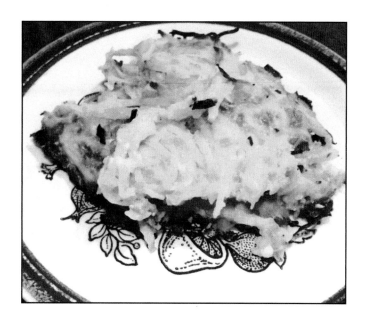

Baked Hash Browns

Prep Time: 10 min.
Cook Time: 50-60 min.
Makes: 10-12 servings

6 c potatoes, peeled and shredded

2 c cheddar cheese, shredded

3/4 c green onions, sliced

1 c milk

1 Tbsp cornstarch

1 tsp chicken base

1 c sour cream

1. Preheat oven to 375°F. In large bowl, mix potatoes, cheddar cheese, and green onions. Put aside.

2. In a separate bowl, combine milk, cornstarch, and chicken base. Add sour cream and mix thoroughly. Stir liquids into potato mixture.

3. Spread evenly in greased 9x13 pan. Bake 50-60 min. or until lightly browned and potatoes are soft.

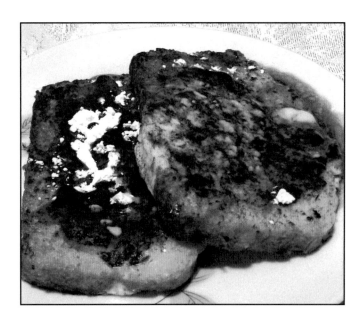

French Toast

Prep Time: 5 min.
Cook Time: 10 min.
Makes: 4-6 slices

1 egg

1/2 c milk

dash salt

1 tsp cinnamon (optional)

4-6 slices yeast or Irish soda bread (p.178-179)

1. In bowl, beat egg, milk, salt, and cinnamon together until blended.

2. Dip each slice of bread in the mixture, making sure to coat both sides. Fry in skillet or on a griddle. Cook both sides until golden brown. Top with powdered sugar or syrup.

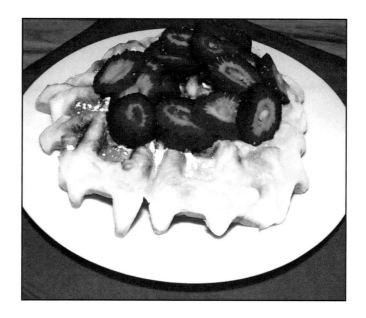

Belgian Waffles

Prep Time: 10 min.

Cook Time: 5-10 min. per waffle

Makes: 4 waffles

1 c all-purpose rice flour blend

2 Tbsp butter

1 large egg

1 c milk

1 tsp vanilla extract

1. In medium bowl, combine rice flour and butter until crumbly. Mix in egg, milk, and vanilla extract.

2. On hot greased waffle iron, add a spoonful of mix in the middle. Press down and cook until desired texture (shorter for softer, longer for crispier). Top with favorite toppings.

Variations: Can add less milk to make mix thicker, more to make it thinner.

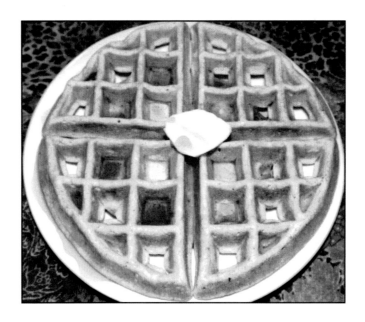

Cinnamon Sugar Waffles

Prep Time: 10 min.

Cook Time: 5-10 min. per waffle

Makes: 4 waffles

I c all-purpose rice flour blend

2 Tbsp butter

I large egg

I c milk

I tsp vanilla

I tsp cinnamon

I Tbsp sugar

1. In medium bowl, combine rice flour and butter until crumbly. Mix in egg, milk, vanilla, cinnamon, and sugar until smooth.

2. In hot greased waffle iron, add mix to middle, press down. Cook until desired texture (shorter for softer, longer for crispier). Top with favorite toppings.

Variations: Can add less milk to make mix thicker, more to make it thinner.

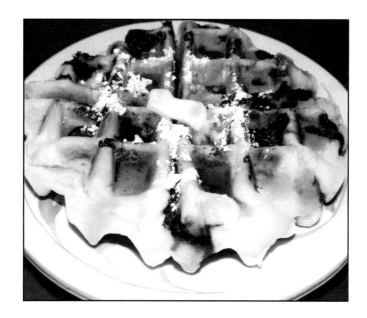

Blueberry Waffles

Prep Time: 10 min.

Cook Time: 5-10 min. per waffle

Makes: 4 waffles

1 c all-purpose rice flour blend

2 Tbsp butter

1 large egg

1 c milk

1 tsp vanilla

1 c blueberries, fresh or frozen

1. In medium bowl, combine rice flour and butter until crumbly. Add egg, milk, and vanilla.

Stir until smooth. Add blueberries and stir until incorporated.

2. In hot greased waffle iron, add mix to middle and press down. Cook until desired texture

(shorter for softer, longer for crispier). Top with favorite toppings.

Variations: Can add less milk to make mix thicker, more to make it thinner.

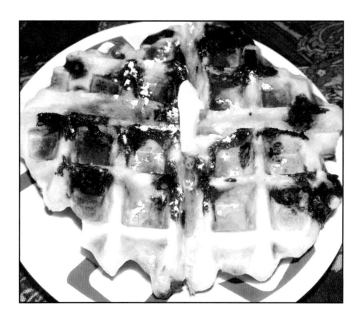

Blueberry Yogurt Waffles

Prep Time: 10 min.

Cook Time: 5-10 min. per waffle

Makes: 4 waffles

1 c all-purpose rice flour blend

2 Tbsp butter

1 c greek or plain yogurt

1 c milk

1 tsp vanilla

1 c blueberries, frozen or fresh

1. In medium bowl, combine rice flour and butter until crumbly. Add yogurt, milk, and vanilla until smooth. Add blueberries and mix well.

2. In hot greased waffle iron, add mix to middle and press down. Cook until desired texture (shorter for softer, longer for crispier). Top with favorite toppings.

Variations: Can add less milk to make mix thicker, more to make it thinner.

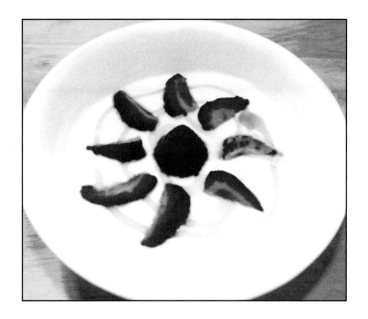

Strawberry Honey Yogurt

Prep Time: 10 min.
Makes: 1 1/2 cups

1 c plain yogurt

1 tsp honey

1/2 c strawberries, sliced

1. In bowl, blend together yogurt and honey.

2. Top with strawberries. Stir until incorporated. Eat cold.

Variations: Can use sugar instead of honey, or for a less sweet taste, leave out honey.

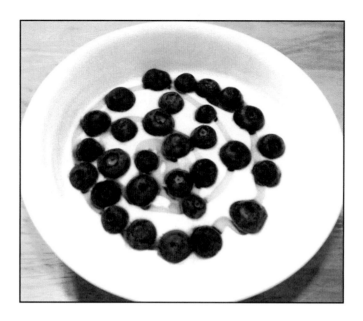

Blueberry Honey Yogurt

Prep Time: 10 min.

Makes: 1 1/4 cups

1 c plain yogurt

1 tsp honey

1/4 c blueberries

1. In bowl, blend together yogurt and honey.

2. Top with blueberries. Stir until incorporated. Eat cold.

Variations: Can use sugar instead of honey, or for a less sweet taste, leave out honey.

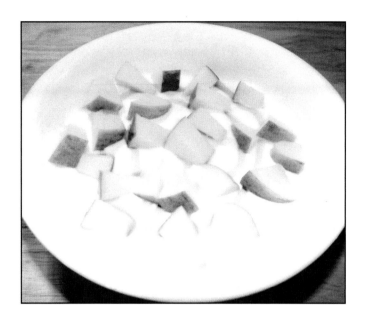

Apple Honey Yogurt

Prep Time: 10 min.

Makes: 1 1/2 cups

1 c plain yogurt

1 tsp honey

1/2 c apples, cored and chopped

1. In bowl, blend together yogurt and honey.

2. Top with apple pieces. Stir until incorporated. Eat cold.

Variations: Can use sugar instead of honey, or for a less sweet taste, leave out honey.

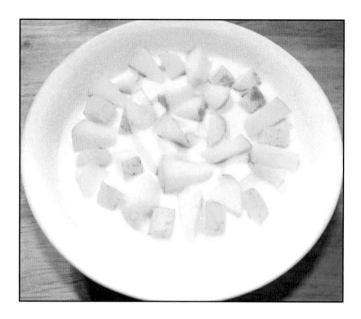

Pear Honey Yogurt

Prep Time: 10 min.

Makes: 1 1/2 cups

1 c plain yogurt

1 tsp honey

1/2 c pears, cored and chopped

1. In bowl, blend together yogurt and honey.

2. Top with pear pieces. Stir until incorporated. Eat cold.

Variations: Can use sugar instead of honey, or for a less sweet taste, leave out honey.

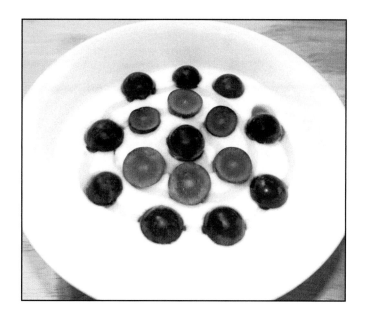

Grape Honey Yogurt

Prep Time: 10 min.

Makes: 1 1/4 cups

1 c plain yogurt

1 tsp honey

1/4 c red grapes, halved

1. In bowl, blend together yogurt and honey.

2. Top with grapes. Blend until incorporated. Serve cold.

Variations: Can use sugar instead of honey, or for a less sweet taste, leave out honey.

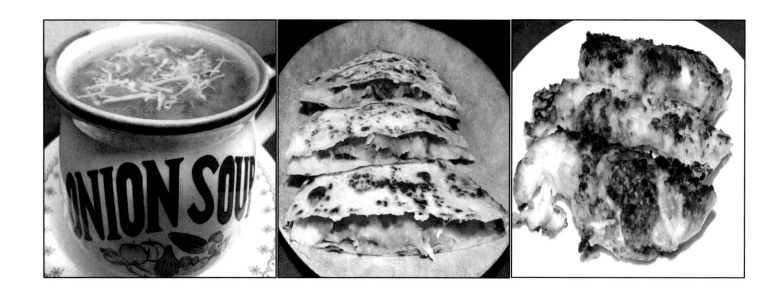

Main Dishes —Lunch

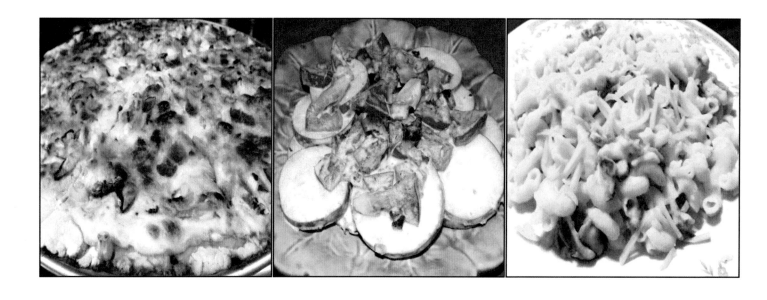

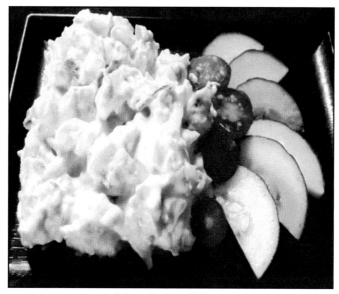

Chicken Salad

Prep Time: 15 min.

Chill Time: 1 hr.

Makes: 3-4 cups

1 c cooked chicken, shredded or cubed

1 tsp salt or seasoning salt

1/2 c mayonnaise

1/2 c onions, chopped

1/4 c sour cream

1/2 c red grapes, halved (optional)

1/2 c apples, cored and cubed (optional)

1. In medium bowl, mix chicken, salt, mayonnaise, onions, and sour cream together until coated.

2. Can add red grapes or apples if desired. Chill for an hour. Serve cold.

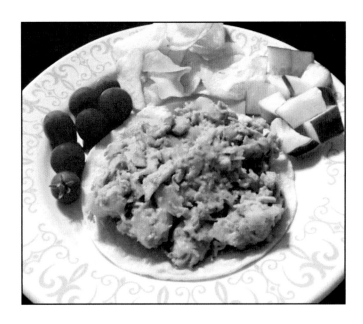

Pulled Pork

Prep Time: 20 min.
Cook Time: 4 hrs.
Makes: 6-8 servings

2-3 lbs pork roast or pork tenderloin

2 c water

salt and pepper to taste

1 tsp onion powder

1/2 c diced onions

2 Tbsp butter

2 Tbsp all-purpose rice flour blend

1. Cut pork into small pieces. Put pork into a slow cooker with water. Season with salt, pepper, and onion powder. Top with diced onions. Turn on high heat and cook until tender.

2. Pull apart with fork. Drain juice into bowl to make brown gravy.

3. In saucepan, add butter. When melted, add rice flour to make a rue. Whisk in the juice and cook until thickened. Add gravy to meat. Serve hot.

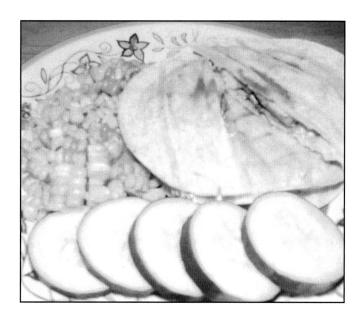

Chicken Fajitas

Prep Time: 5 min.

Cook Time: 5-10 min. per sandwich

Makes: 4 sandwiches

2-3 Tbsp sour cream

8 white or yellow corn tortillas

2 tsp oregano or Italian seasoning

I sprig green onions, chopped

I piece cooked chicken breast, sliced

1/2 c shredded cheese

1. Spread sour cream on one tortilla shell. Sprinkle on some oregano and green onion. Add a few slices of chicken in the middle. Sprinkle on shredded cheese and top with another tortilla shell.

2. Place in pan or on grill. Flip when it starts to brown. Cook until the cheese is melted. Repeat for the other sandwiches.

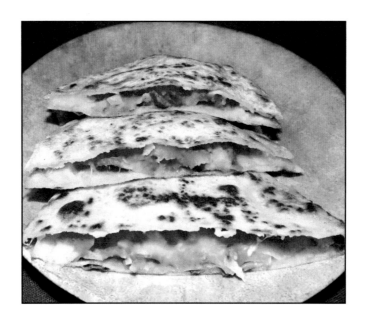

Bacon Sandwich

Prep Time: 5 min.

Cook Time: 5-10 min.

Makes: 2 sandwiches

2 slices bacon

4 white or yellow corn tortillas

2 slices Monterey Jack cheese

2 slices cheddar cheese

1 sprig green onions, chopped

1 Tbsp mayonnaise

1 tomato, sliced

1. Cook bacon until crispy. On one tortilla, layer on 1 slice Monterey Jack cheese and 1 slice cheddar cheese. Add 1/2 sprig chopped green onion and 1 slice bacon.

2. On another tortilla, spread 1/2 Tbsp mayonnaise. Stick together and fry up with the cheese side down. When cheese is melted, separate off the top and place some tomato slices on the bacon. Replace top and repeat for the second sandwich. Do not cook the tomato.

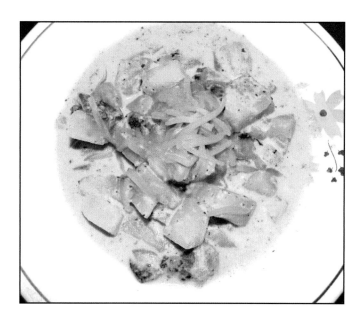

Potato Soup

Prep Time: 10 min.

Cook Time: 30 min.

Makes: 3-4 servings

4 slices bacon, cut into pieces

1 c onions, chopped

3 c potatoes, peeled and diced

3 c milk

1 tsp salt

1/2 tsp pepper

shredded cheese to top (optional)

1. In a pan, fry bacon and onions, stirring for 3 min. Add potatoes and cook slightly until softened.

2. Add milk, salt, and pepper. Cook until potatoes are tender, about 10 min. Serve with shredded cheese on top.

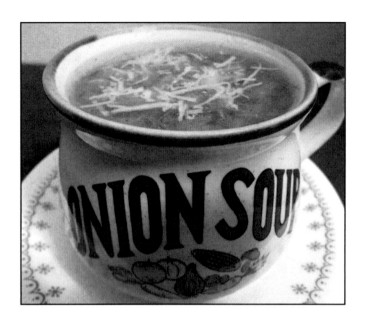

French Onion Soup

Prep Time: 5 min.

Cook Time: 20-25 min.

Makes: 4 servings

1/4 c salted butter

2 c onions, quartered and sliced thin

1 Tbsp all-purpose rice flour blend

4 c beef broth (p.185)

salt and pepper to taste (optional)

white cheese (shredded or sliced)

homemade bread or crackers (optional)

1. In a 4 quart pan, melt butter. Add onions and cook until lightly browned. Dust with rice flour, stirring until onions are browned.

2. Add beef broth, salt, and pepper. Cover and reduce heat to low. Cook 15-20 min.

3. Serve with white cheese (shredded or sliced) and homemade bread or crackers.

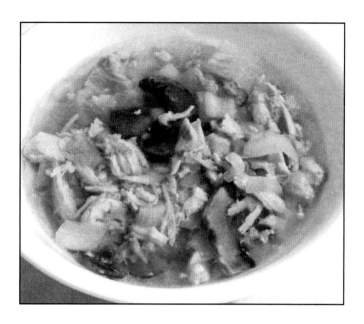

Chicken and Mushroom Soup

Prep Time: 15 min.

Cook Time: 30 min.

Makes: 3-4 servings

1/2 c potatoes, peeled and chopped

1/2 c celery, sliced

1 c cabbage, chopped fine

1/2 c onions, diced

1 c raw chicken, cubed

1/2 c mushrooms, sliced

2 c chicken broth or stock (p.184)

1 Tbsp chicken base (optional)

1/2 tsp onion powder

salt and pepper to taste

1. In pot, add potatoes, celery, cabbage, onions, chicken, mushrooms, chicken broth, chicken base, onion powder, salt, and pepper.

2. Cook until vegetables are tender. Serve hot.

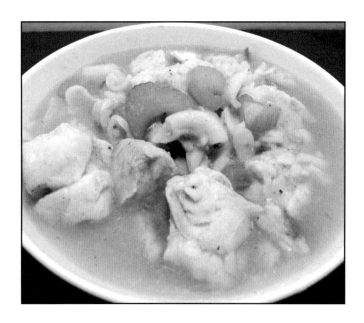

Chicken Noodle Soup

Prep Time: 10 min.

Cook Time: 30 min.

Makes: 4 servings

2 c cooked chicken, cubed

3 c water mixed with 3 Tbsp chicken base

OR 3 c chicken broth (p.184)

1 c onions, diced

1 c celery, sliced

salt and pepper to taste

2 c cooked corn pasta

1. In a large pot, mix together chicken, chicken base mixture, onions, celery, salt, and pepper.

2. Cook on high until celery is tender. Add noodles and cook 5 more min.

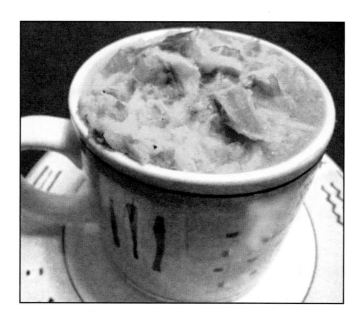

Zucchini Soup

Prep Time: 20 min.

Cook Time: 30 min.

Makes: 4 servings

2 c zucchini, peeled and cubed

1 c onions, diced

1 1/2 c chicken, cooked and cubed

2 tsp chicken base

2 c chicken broth (p.184)

1/2 c uncooked rice

1 tsp salt

1/2 tsp pepper

2 c water

1. In a large pot, combine zucchini, onions, chicken, chicken base, chicken broth, and rice. Add salt, pepper, and water.

2. Boil soup 30 min. or until vegetables are tender and rice is cooked. Eat hot.

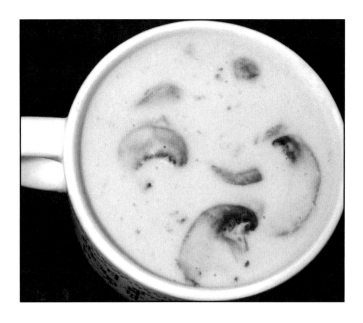

Cream of Mushroom Soup

Prep Time: 5 min.
Cook Time: 20-25 min.
Makes: 2-3 servings

2 Tbsp butter, salted

2 Tbsp canola oil

1 8-oz pkg mushrooms, sliced

2 Tbsp all-purpose rice flour blend

3 c milk

1 tsp seasoning salt

1/2 c half and half

1. Melt butter and oil in large pot. Add mushrooms. Cook until mushrooms darken. Dust with rice flour and cook until golden brown.

2. Add milk, 1 cup at a time, seasoning salt, and half and half. Stir; cook on high for 5 min. Turn to medium heat for 10 min. Let stand 5 min. and serve.

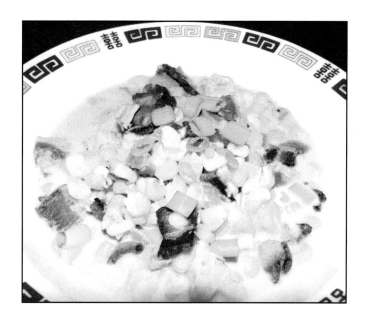

Corn and Bacon Chowder

Prep Time: 25 min.

Cook Time: 25 min.

Makes: 2-3 servings

4-5 slices bacon, chopped

1 c onions, chopped

1/2 c celery, chopped

2 c corn, cooked cob corn or frozen thawed

1 Tbsp chicken base

1 1/2 - 2 c whole milk

salt and pepper to taste

chopped green onions for serving (optional)

1. In a large skillet, cook bacon on medium heat until it sizzles. Add onions and celery. Cook until lightly browned.

2. Add corn, chicken base, milk, salt, and pepper. Cook 5-10 min. or until corn is cooked. Serve with green onions on top.

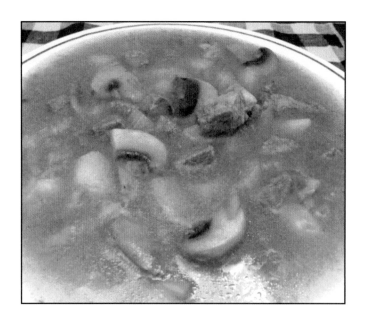

Beef Stew

Prep Time: 25 min.
Cook Time: 65 min.
Makes: 4-5 servings

1 Tbsp olive oil
1 Tbsp butter, salted
2 c beef, cubed
1 tsp salt
1/2 tsp pepper
1 tsp onion powder
1 tsp seasoning salt
4 c water
1 c onions, cubed
1 c celery, sliced
2 c potatoes, peeled and cubed
2 c mushrooms, sliced
1/4 c cold water mixed with 2 Tbsp cornstarch

1. In a skillet, heat the olive oil and brown together the butter, beef, salt, pepper, onion powder, and seasoning salt. Put in a large pot, rinsing the skillet with some of the water and adding it to the pot.

2. Add onions, celery, potatoes, mushrooms, and the rest of the water. Cover and cook on medium heat for 15 min.

3. Reduce heat to low for 45 min. and cook until the meat is tender. Return to high heat and add the cornstarch mixture. Cook for 5 minutes until the stew thickens. Serve hot.

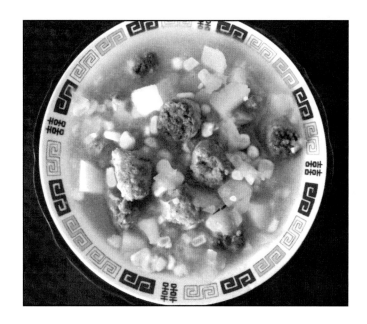

Sausage Stew

Prep Time: 20 min.

Cook Time: 30 min.

Makes: 2-3 servings

1 c sliced bratwurst or pork sausage

1 tsp onion powder

1 tsp salt

1/2 tsp pepper

1 c zucchini, peeled and cubed

1 c onions, chopped

1 c corn, fresh or frozen

1 c potatoes, peeled and cubed

2 c water

1. Brown bratwurst slices in skillet. In pot, add onion powder, salt, pepper, bratwurst, zucchini, onions, corn, potatoes, and water.

2. Cook 20 min. or until vegetables are soft. Serve hot.

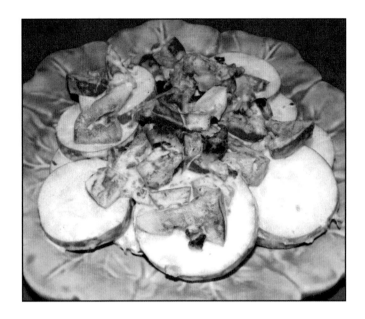

Bacon Tomato Cucumber Salad

Prep Time: 15 min.

Makes: 2 cups

1-2 cucumbers, sliced

1 tomato, chopped

1-2 Tbsp mayonnaise

salt and pepper to taste

3 slices bacon, cooked and crumbled

1. In bowl, add cucumbers, tomatoes, mayonnaise, salt, and pepper. Stir.

2. Add crumbled bacon. Mix until incorporated. Serve chilled.

Variations: Can use hard boiled eggs instead of bacon, or cooked chicken breast cubes.

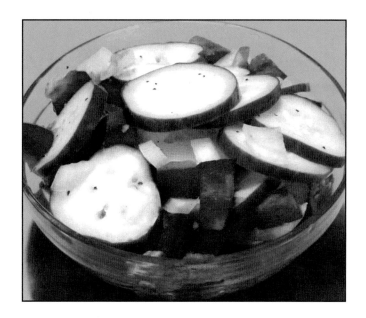

Cucumber Onion Tomato Salad

Prep Time: 10 min.

Chill Time: 1-2 hrs.

Makes: 6-8 servings

3 tomatoes, diced

3 cucumbers, sliced

1 onion, diced

1/2 c apple cider vinegar

1/4 c olive oil

1 tsp pepper

2 Tbsp sugar

2 tsp salt

1. In bowl, mix together tomatoes, cucumbers, and onions. Add apple cider vinegar and olive oil; stir until coated.

2. Sprinkle on pepper, sugar, and salt. Chill in refrigerator 1-2 hrs. Serve cold.

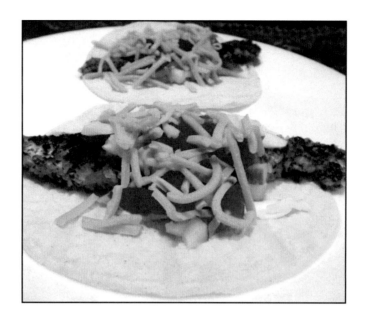

Soft Shell Chicken Tacos

Prep Time: 15 min.

Cook Time: 10 min.

Makes: 4 tacos

2 strips chicken breast

2 Tbsp onion ranch dressing mix (p.2)

4 white or yellow corn tortillas

1/4 c onions, diced

1/4 c cabbage, shredded

1/4 c tomatoes, diced

1/4 c cheese, shredded

1. Cut chicken breast strips in half the long way. Press into onion ranch dressing mix and grill on both sides.

2. Warm the tortillas in the microwave for 10 seconds to loosen them up. Add cooked chicken, onions, cabbage, tomatoes, and cheese to each tortilla. Serve warm.

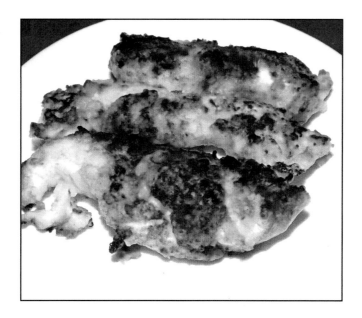

Balsamic Chicken Breast Strips

Prep Time: 5 min.

Cook Time: 15 min.

Makes: 8-12 strips

1-2 chicken breasts, sliced into strips

1/3 c olive oil

1-2 tsp blueberry balsamic vinegar

1. In a pan, add chicken and olive oil. Fry chicken until white on both sides.

2. Drizzle blueberry balsamic over chicken pieces. Reduce heat, turning until coated.

3. Cook down sauce, watching that it doesn't burn. Serve hot.

Variations: Can use regular balsamic vinegar sauce if blueberry is unavailable.

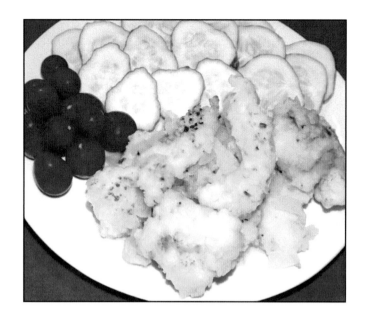

Homestyle Fried Chicken

Prep Time: 10 min.

Cook Time: 10 min.

Makes: 8-12 strips

1/2 c all-purpose rice flour blend

1 tsp seasoning salt

1/2 tsp black pepper

2 Tbsp canola oil

1-2 pieces chicken breasts, cut into strips

1 egg, beaten

1. In medium bowl, mix rice flour with seasoning salt and black pepper. Heat canola oil in saucepan over medium heat.

2. Dip each chicken strip into egg mixture, then rice flour mixture, coating both sides. Place in saucepan and cook with lid until golden brown on both sides and white in the middle.

3. Eat hot. Can dip in dipping sauce.

Variations: Can add 1 tsp onion flakes if desired.

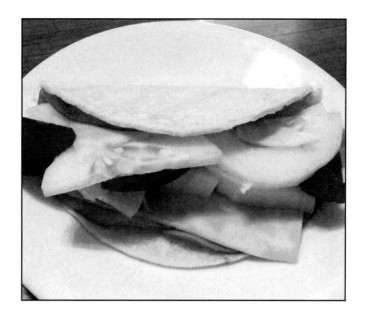

Ham and Cheese Tortilla Rolls

Prep Time: 15 min.

Makes: 2 rolls

1/3 c cheddar cheese, shredded

1 Tbsp mayonnaise

2 tsp sour cream

1/4 c corn

2 white or yellow corn tortillas

2 slices ham

1. In bowl, combine cheese, mayonnaise, sour cream, and corn. Stir well.

2. On a tortilla, place one slice of ham. Spread 1/2 of the corn mixture over ham. Roll up and serve.

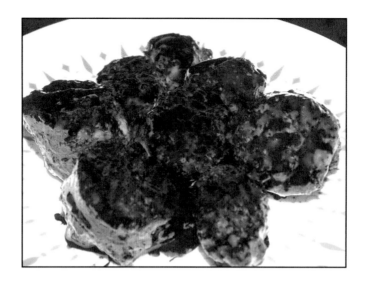

Blueberry Balsamic Bratwurst

Prep Time: 5 min.

Cook Time: 15 min.

Makes: 3-4 servings

1/3 c olive oil

4 brats, cut into 1/2-in. pieces

2 Tbsp blueberry balsamic vinegar

1. Heat olive oil in a skillet on medium heat. Add brat pieces. Cook for 2-3 min on each side. Drizzle with blueberry balsamic.

2. Cook 3 minutes, then flip and cook for 2 more min. Use remaining sauce to make a glaze. Serve hot.

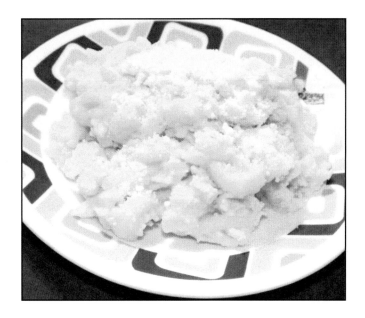

Slow Cooker Mac and Cheese

Prep Time: 20 min.

Cook Time: 1 hr. 30 min.

Makes: 4 servings

1 1/2 c whole milk or half and half

1/4 c melted cooled butter

3 eggs

1/2 tsp salt

4 c cooked corn macaroni

3 c shredded cheese

parmesan cheese to top (optional)

1. Whisk together milk, butter, eggs, and salt. Add to crockpot. Stir in corn macaroni and shredded cheese.

2. Cook on high 1 hr. 30 min. Serve warm with a sprinkle of parmesan if desired.

Variations: Bake in oven 1 hour at 375°F in greased 9x13 pan.

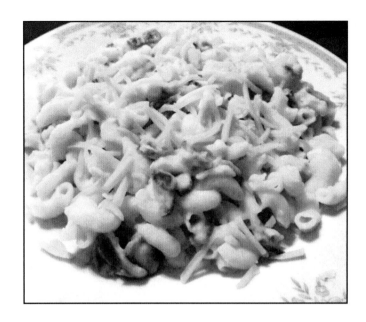

Bacon Macaroni and Cheese

Prep Time: 15 min.

Cook Time: 15 min.

Makes: 4 servings

1 c cheddar cheese, shredded

2 Tbsp butter

1/2 c milk

2 c cooked corn elbow noodles

6 slices bacon, chopped and cooked

salt and pepper to taste

1. Combine cheddar cheese, butter, and milk in saucepan. Heat until boiling.

2. Stir in cooked elbow noodles, bacon pieces, salt, and pepper. Stir until incorporated.

Variations: Add whole milk or half and half to make creamier.

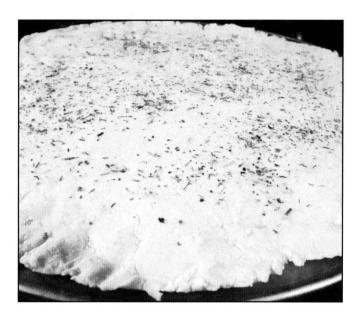

Pizza Dough

Prep Time: 25 min.

Cook Time: 30 min.

Makes: 1 large pizza or 2 small pizzas

1 Tbsp yeast

1 c warm water

2 tsp sugar

1/2 c butter

3 c all-purpose rice flour blend

1 egg

1 tsp salt

1 Tbsp Italian seasoning (optional)

1. Preheat oven to 400°F. Add yeast to warm water and sugar. Let yeast raise 5 min. In bowl, crumble in butter into the rice flour. Add yeast mixture, egg, and salt.

2. Mix until dough texture forms, adding more flour as needed to make less sticky. Spread onto greased pizza pan and let sit 10 min. Cook in oven for 10 min. Sprinkle with Italian seasoning. Use to make pizza.

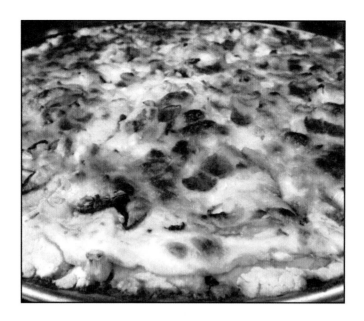

Cream Cheese Spread Pizza

Prep Time: 20 min.
Cook Time: 15-18 min.
Makes: 8 servings

1 homemade pizza crust (p.87)

1 Tbsp butter, melted

1 pkg (8 oz) cream cheese, softened

2 Tbsp parmesan cheese

salt to taste

1 Tbsp oregano

2 c cheese, pizza blend

1 c mushrooms, chopped

1 c green onions, chopped

1 tomato, dehydrated and shredded (optional)

1. Preheat oven to 400°F. On greased pizza pan, spread out dough. Bake 10 min; remove.

2. In medium bowl, combine melted butter, cream cheese, parmesan cheese, salt, and oregano. Blend until smooth. Spread over pizza crust.

3. Top evenly with cheese. Add mushrooms, green onions, and dehydrated tomatoes on top. Cook 15-18 min. or until crust is cooked through and cheese is melted. Serve hot.

Variations: Can use a diced tomato if you don't have dehydrated ones. Put them on after the pizza is cooked.

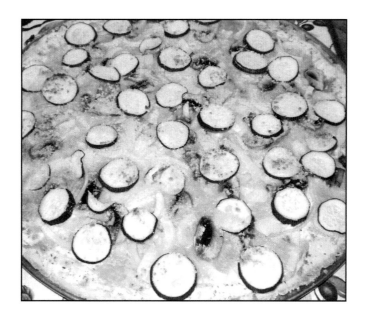

Three Cheese Garden Pizza

Prep Time: 20 min.

Cook Time: 15-18 min.

Makes: 8 servings

1 homemade pizza crust (p.87)

1 tsp Italian seasoning

1 c shredded mozzarella cheese

1 c shredded cheddar cheese

1 medium zucchini, thinly sliced

1 small onion, sliced

1 c fresh mushrooms, sliced

1/4 c shredded parmesan cheese

1. Preheat oven to 400°F. On greased pizza pan, spread out dough. Bake 10 min; remove.

2. Sprinkle on Italian seasoning. Add mozzarella and cheddar cheeses. Top with zucchini, onions, and mushrooms. Sprinkle with parmesan cheese. Bake 15-18 min. Cut and serve hot.

Variations: Can add the cream cheese pizza spread to crust if desired (see recipe).

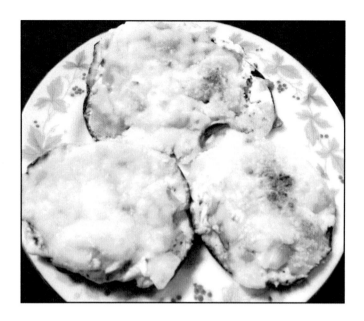

Eggplant Pizza

Prep Time: 50 min.

Cook Time: 35 min.

Makes: 4 servings

1 **eggplant**

1 **Tbsp salt**

1 **pkg (8 oz) cream cheese, softened**

1/2 **c sour cream**

1 **Tbsp Italian seasoning**

2 **Tbsp olive oil**

1/3 **c parmesan cheese**

1/3 **c mozzarella cheese**

1. Preheat oven to 375°F. Cut off ends of eggplant and slice into pieces 1/4-in. thick. Lay on paper towel and sprinkle salt over the pieces. Let sit for 30 min.

2. In small bowl, mix cream cheese and sour cream with 1 tsp Italian seasoning. Set aside.

3. Wipe eggplants dry with paper towel. On greased baking pan, layer eggplant slices across the bottom. Brush with olive oil, sprinkle with remaining Italian seasoning. Roast 20 min., then spread on sauce. Top with favorite pizza toppings and sprinkle with cheeses. Cook 15 min.

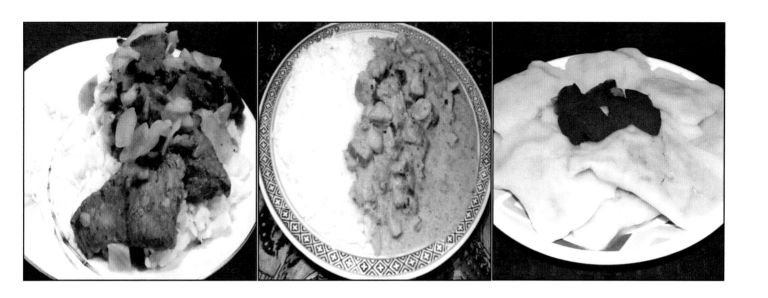

Main Dishes —Dinner

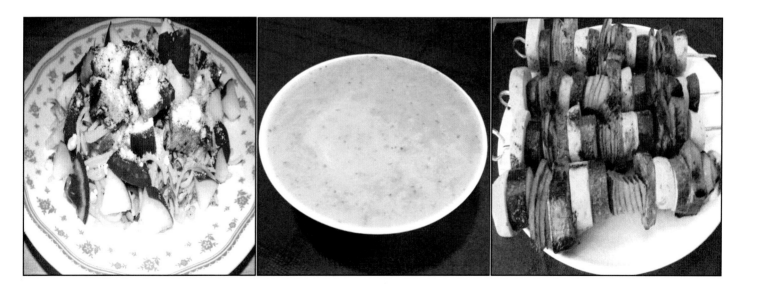

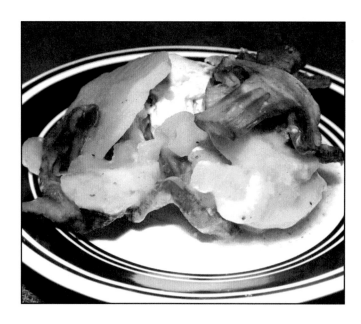

Crock Pot Chicken

Prep Time: 20 min.
Cook Time: 2 hrs.
Makes: 4 servings

2 c chicken breast, cubed

1 c celery, sliced

1 c potatoes, peeled and sliced

1 c onions, diced

1 c mushrooms, sliced

1 tsp salt

1/2 tsp pepper

1 Tbsp butter

2 c cold water mixed with 2 Tbsp cornstarch

2 Tbsp chicken base (or 2 c cold chicken stock mixed with 2 Tbsp cornstarch)

1. In crock pot, layer in chicken, celery, potatoes, onions, and mushrooms. Add salt and pepper.

2. In saucepan, place butter and melt. Stir in cornstarch mixture and chicken base. Cook until thickened, stirring occasionally.

3. Add sauce to crockpot. Cook 2 hrs. on high until vegetables are tender.

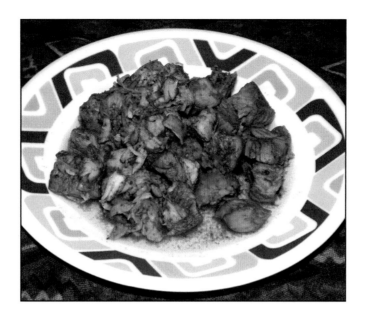

Sweet Crock Pot Chicken

Prep Time: 10 min.
Cook Time: 6-8 hrs.
Makes: 3-4 servings

2 lbs chicken breast, cubed
1/4 c balsamic vinegar
1/2 c brown sugar
2 Tbsp mirin or rice vinegar
1 tsp salt
1 Tbsp honey

1. In crock pot, combine chicken, balsamic vinegar, brown sugar, mirin, salt, and honey. Stir until chicken is coated.

2. Cook on high 3-4 hrs. until chicken is cooked through. Serve hot.

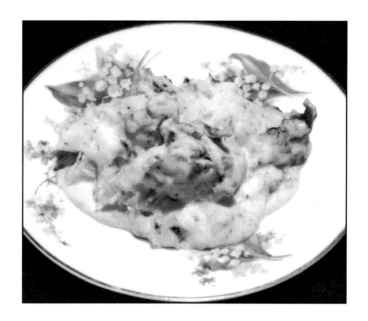

Slow Cooker Cracked Chicken

Prep Time: 15 min.

Cook Time: 4 hrs.

Makes: 4 servings

4 pieces boneless, skinless chicken breasts

1 pkg (8 oz) cream cheese

2 Tbsp ranch dressing mix (p.2)

1 c bacon, cooked and crumbled

1. In a slow cooker, combine chicken, cream cheese, and ranch dressing mix. Cook on high for 4 hrs. or until chicken comes apart easily.

2. Stir chicken, breaking it apart. Add bacon on top, stirring to incorporate. Serve warm.

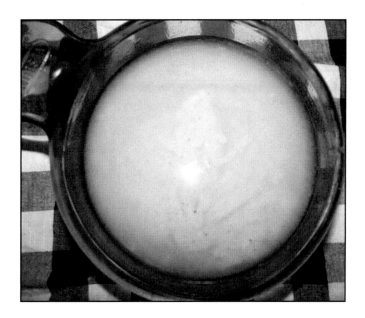

Chicken Barbecue Sauce

Prep Time: 15 min.
Makes: 1-2 cups

1 egg
1 c canola or olive oil
2 Tbsp vinegar
1 Tbsp chicken base
1 tsp salt
1 tsp pepper

1. In bowl, beat eggs. Pour in oil and vinegar. Blend until incorporated.

2. Sprinkle on chicken base, salt, and pepper. Stir until blended. Brush on chicken and cook as desired.

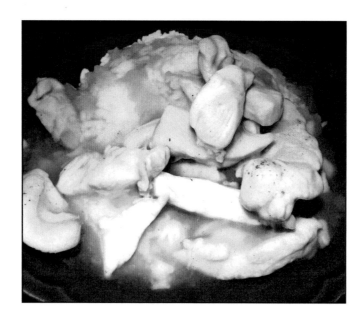

Mock Orange Chicken

Prep Time: 15 min.
Cook Time: 20 min.
Makes: 3-4 servings

2 Tbsp canola oil

4 chicken breasts, cut into strips

salt and pepper to taste

1/2 c onions, diced

1/4 c white wine vinegar

2 Tbsp cornstarch mixed with 1 c cold water

3/4 c honey

cooked rice to plate

1. In skillet, heat canola oil. Add chicken breast strips and season with salt and pepper. Add onions. Cook until chicken is white.

2. Add vinegar, cornstarch mixture, and honey. Stir constantly to make sure it won't stick. Cook until sauce thickens and coats chicken. Serve hot over rice.

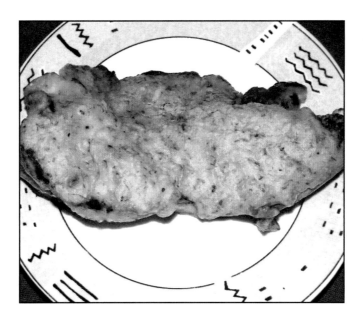

Mustard Glazed Chicken

Prep Time: 15 min.

Cook Time: 20 min.

Makes: 2 servings

2 Tbsp onion ranch mix (p.2)

4 Tbsp butter, softened

1 tsp yellow mustard

1/2 c half and half

1/4 c all-purpose rice flour blend

2 chicken breasts, whole or in strips

1. Preheat oven to 375°F. In bowl, combine ranch mix, 2 Tbsp butter, mustard, half and half, and rice flour. In skillet, melt the remaining 2 Tbsp butter. Place chicken in skillet and sear 5 min. on both sides.

2. Remove from pan. Coat both sides of chicken with mustard mixture. Place chicken in greased baking pan. Bake 20 in. until cooked through. Remove from pan and serve with favorite side.

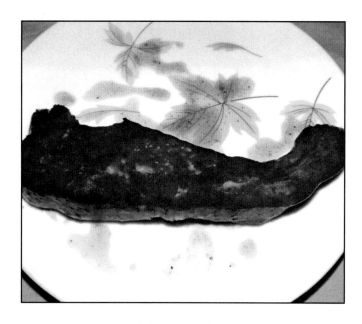

Honey Mustard Chicken

Prep Time: 5 min.

Cook Time: 15 min.

Makes: 4 servings

4 chicken breasts, whole or in strips

salt and pepper to taste

1 Tbsp yellow mustard

1 Tbsp honey

1 Tbsp apple cider vinegar

1 tsp onion powder

1. In skillet, add chicken, salt, and pepper. In bowl, add mustard, honey, vinegar, and onion powder. Mix until incorporated.

2. Turn chicken over and glaze with sauce. Cook until white in the center.

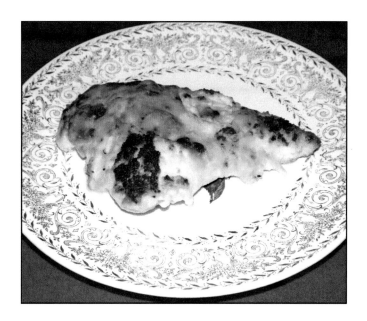

Swiss Chicken Bake

Prep Time: 15 min.

Cook Time: 1 hr.

Makes: 4-6 servings

4-6 boneless, skinless chicken breasts

6-8 slices Swiss cheese

1/2 c mayonnaise

1/2 c sour cream

3/4 c parmesan cheese (divided)

1/2 tsp salt

1/2 tsp pepper

1. Preheat oven to 375°F. Place chicken in greased 9x13 pan. Top with Swiss cheese. Set aside.

2. In bowl, mix together mayonnaise, sour cream, 1/2 c parmesan cheese, salt, and pepper. Spread over chicken and sprinkle on remaining parmesan cheese. Bake 1 hr. until golden brown.

Variations: Can use mozzarella cheese in place of Swiss.

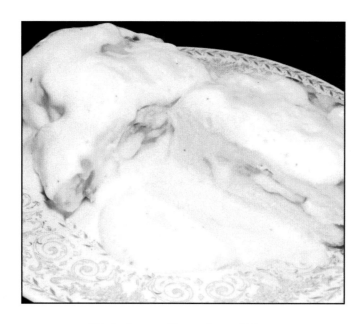

Chicken Cordon Bleu

Prep Time: 15 min.

Cook Time: 40 min.

Makes: 6 servings

6 chicken breasts, sliced open

6 slices Swiss cheese

6 slices ham

3 Tbsp all-purpose rice flour blend

6 Tbsp butter

I Tbsp cornstarch mixed with I c heavy cream

I tsp chicken base

1. Place a cheese and ham slice in each breast within 1/2-in. of edge. Fold edges of chicken over filling, securing with toothpicks. Coat each chicken piece with rice flour.

2. Heat butter in skillet. Cook chicken until brown on both sides. Reduce and cover 30 min. or until fully cooked. Remove toothpicks.

3. In saucepan, blend cornstarch with cream. Add chicken base and cook until thick. Top chicken with sauce. Serve warm.

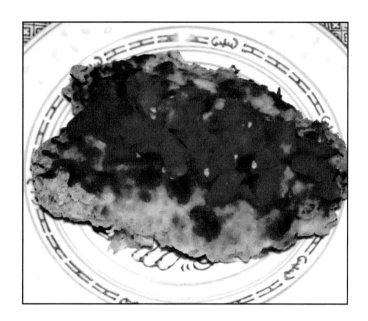

Chicken Parmesan

Prep Time: 20 min.
Cook Time: 15-20 min.
Makes: 4 servings

2 eggs, beaten

1/2 c parmesan cheese

4 boneless, skinless chicken breast halves

1 c olive oil for frying

1 c Italian style shredded cheese

1 Tbsp olive oil

1/2 c fresh tomatoes, chopped

<u>Rice Flour Mix:</u>

1 tsp salt

2 c all-purpose rice flour blend

1/2 tsp pepper

1/2 c grated parmesan

1 tsp Italian seasoning

1. Preheat oven to 450°F. Mix rice flour mix and 1/2 c parmesan cheese, set aside. Coat chicken in rice flour mix, evenly coating both sides. Dip in egg batter. Press in more rice flour mix. Set aside.

2. Heat 1 c olive oil in skillet. Cook chicken until golden on each side. Place in greased baking dish. Top with cheese and 1 Tbsp olive oil.

3. Bake 15-20 min. until no longer pink. Take out and top with fresh tomatoes.

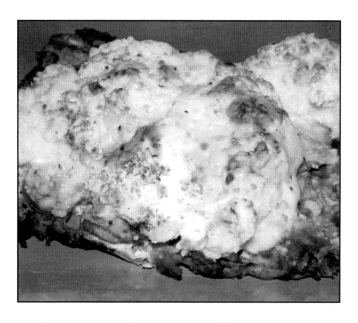

Breaded Chicken & Mushrooms

Prep Time: 15 min.

Cook Time: 45 min.

Makes: 8 servings

1 egg

salt and pepper to taste

1/2 c parmesan cheese

1 c all-purpose rice flour blend

1/4 c butter, melted

1 lb. fresh mushrooms, sliced

8 boneless, skinless chicken breast halves

1. Preheat oven to 375°F. Beat egg with salt and pepper. In separate bowl, mix parmesan cheese with rice flour. Pour 2/3 butter into a 9x13 baking pan, coating it. Spread mushrooms evenly on the bottom.

2. Dip each chicken piece into the egg mixture, then the rice flour mixture until coated. Place on top of mushrooms. Drizzle remaining butter over chicken. Bake 45 min. until golden brown.

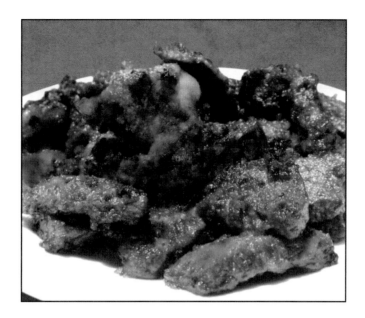

Round Steak

Prep Time: 5 min.

Cook Time: 10 min.

Makes: 4 servings

2 Tbsp olive oil for frying

2 lbs round steak

1/2 c red onion marinade (p.104)

1. Cut steak into pieces. In skillet, add oil and grill steak 4 min. Flip and top with marinade.

2. Cook 4 min. or until done and sauce has reduced in pan. Serve hot.

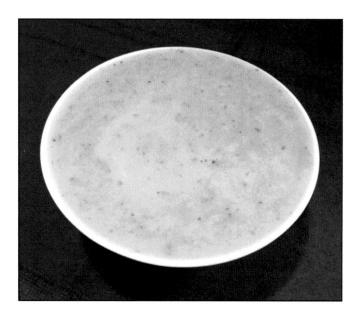

Red Onion Marinade

Prep Time: 5 min.

Makes: 1 1/2 cups

1 c red onions, sliced

1/4 c red wine vinegar

1/2 c olive oil

2 Tbsp brown sugar

1. In food processor, combine onions, vinegar, oil, and sugar.

2. Pulsate into a sauce. Use on meat or over salad.

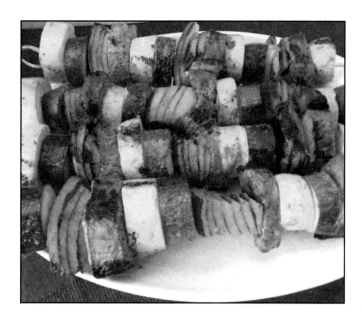

Summer Kabobs

Prep Time: 15 min.
Cook Time: 20-25 min.
Makes: 6-8 kabobs

1 c beef cubes

1 c red onion wedges

1 zucchini, sliced 1/2-in. thick

1 yellow squash, sliced 1/2-in. thick

1/4 c olive oil

1/2 tsp salt

1/2 tsp pepper

1 tsp seasoning salt

1 tsp onion powder

1. On skewers, alternate beef cubes, onion wedges, zucchini slices, and yellow squash slices.

In bowl, combine oil, salt, pepper, seasoning salt, and onion powder. Brush on oil mixture.

2. Grill until steak is thoroughly cooked. Serve hot or over white rice.

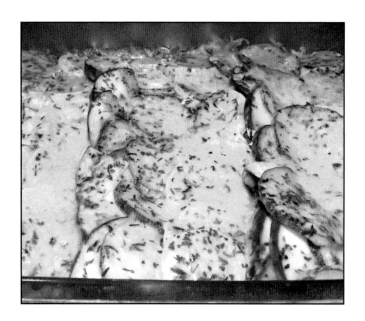

Ratatouille

Prep Time: 45 min.
Cook Time: 45 min.
Makes: 1 pan

1 small eggplant, sliced thin

4 Tbsp olive oil (divided)

2 c chopped meat (beef, pork, or chicken)

1/2 onion, chopped

1/2 c sour cream

salt and pepper to taste

1 yellow summer squash, sliced thin

1 zucchini, sliced thin

1 tsp thyme

1 tsp basil

2 c cheese, shredded

1. Preheat oven to 375°F. Lightly salt each side of eggplant slices, drying on a paper towel for 20 min. Heat 1 Tbsp olive oil in skillet. Sauté meat and onions until browned.

2. In medium bowl, combine meat, onions, sour cream, and 1 Tbsp olive oil. Mix well. Season with salt and pepper. Spread on the bottom of a greased 9x13 pan.

3. Lightly coat sliced veggies in 1 Tbsp olive oil. Arrange in alternating layers. Drizzle on remaining olive oil. Season with salt, pepper, thyme, basil, and shredded cheese. Cover with foil and bake 45 min. until tender.

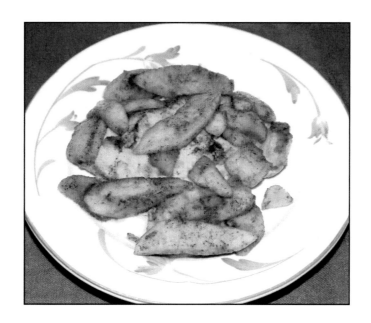

Cinnamon Apple Pork Chops

Prep Time: 5 min.

Cook Time: 15 min.

Makes: 2 servings

2 Tbsp olive oil

2 pork chops

salt and pepper to taste

2 apples, sliced and cored

1 Tbsp brown sugar

1 Tbsp butter

1/2 tsp cinnamon

1. In skillet, heat oil. Add pork chops and season with salt and pepper. Flip and cook through. Remove from pan.

2. In skillet, combine apple slices, brown sugar, butter, and cinnamon. Sauté until golden brown.

3. Spoon over pork chops and serve hot.

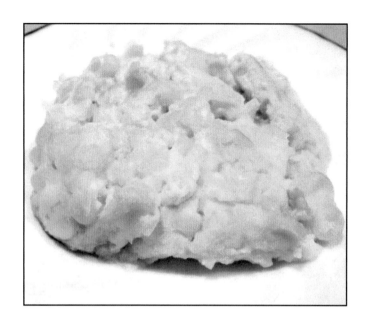

Corn Bake

Prep Time: 20 min.

Cook Time: 25 min.

Makes: 6 servings

2 Tbsp butter

1 Tbsp cornmeal

1 c milk

2 c corn

1/4 c mayonnaise

1/2 c sharp cheddar cheese

1 egg, lightly beaten

1. Preheat oven to 350°F. In saucepan, combine butter, cornmeal, and milk until thickened. In large bowl, combine corn, mayonnaise, cheese, cornmeal mixture, and eggs. Mix well.

2. Place in greased 9x9 baking pan. Bake 25 min. until set and browned.

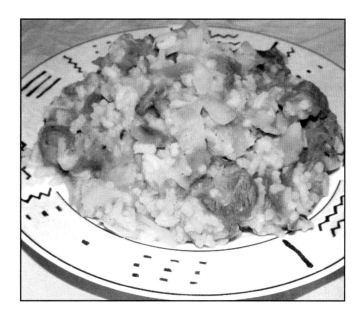

Spanish Cabbage Dish

Prep Time: 20 min.

Cook Time: 25 min.

Makes: 4-6 servings

2 Tbsp butter

1 c onions, chopped

2 c cabbage, cubed

2 c cooked beef cubes

1/4 tsp crushed red pepper

1/4 tsp curry powder (optional)

1 tsp seasoning salt

1/4 tsp black pepper

3 c rice, cooked

2 c beef broth (p.185)

1. In skillet, melt butter. Sauté onions and cabbage until lightly brown. Set aside.

2. Place beef in skillet. Sprinkle on red pepper, curry powder, seasoning salt, and black pepper. Add cooked vegetables and rice to skillet. Pour in beef broth. Cook until thickened. Serve hot.

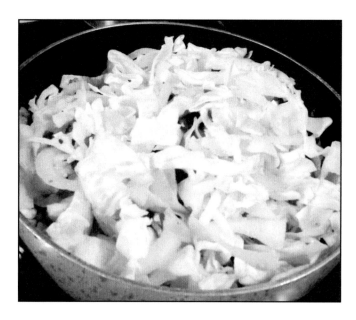

Easy Stir Fry

Prep Time: 15 min.

Cook Time: 20 min.

Makes: 4 servings

1/2 head of cabbage, sliced thin

1 pkg (8 oz) fresh diced mushrooms

1 onion, sliced into strips

1/4 c olive oil

1/2 tsp onion powder

cooked white rice

1. Mix cabbage, mushrooms, and onions together in bowl. In skillet, add olive oil and vegetables. Sprinkle with onion powder.

2. Cover and cook on medium heat for 20 min., stirring occasionally.

3. When vegetables are tender and golden brown, remove from heat. Serve over rice.

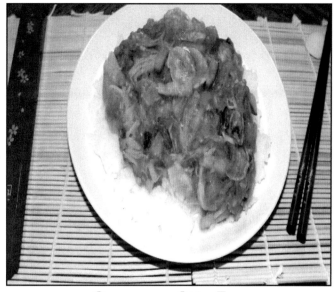

Summer Stir Fry

Prep Time: 20 min.

Cook Time: 30 min.

Makes: 4-6 servings

1/4 c olive oil

1 yellow summer squash, cut in circles

1 zucchini, cut into thin strips

5 large mushrooms, sliced

1/2 onion, sliced long

3 sprigs green onions, diced

1 c fresh or boiled cabbage, sliced

2 c beef or pork roast, with drippings

salt and pepper to taste

1/2 c cornstarch mixed with 1 c cold water

1 Tbsp balsamic vinegar

1. Heat olive oil in skillet. Add veggies and beef. Sprinkle with salt and pepper. Cover.

2. When almost completely cooked, add cornstarch mix and balsamic vinegar. Stir until thickened and cooked through. Serve over rice.

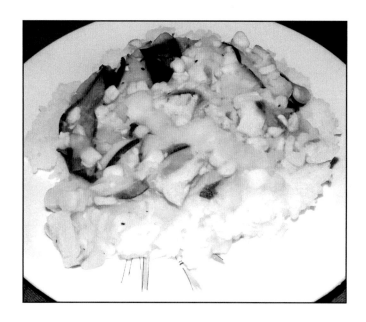

Zucchini Corn Stir Fry

Prep Time: 15 min.
Cook Time: 30 min.
Makes: 2-3 servings

1 Tbsp butter

1 zucchini, julienned skin and diced innards

1 onion, quartered and sliced thin

1 piece cooked chicken breast, diced

1/2 Tbsp sugar

salt and pepper to taste

2 c corn, fresh or frozen

1 tsp chicken base

2 tsp cornstarch mixed with 1 c cold water

cooked white rice to plate

1. Melt butter in skillet. Add zucchini, onions, and chicken to pan. Sprinkle with sugar, salt, pepper, and corn to top. Cover and cook until tender.

2. Mix chicken base and cornstarch mixture together. Pour in pan. Stir until thickened. Serve over rice.

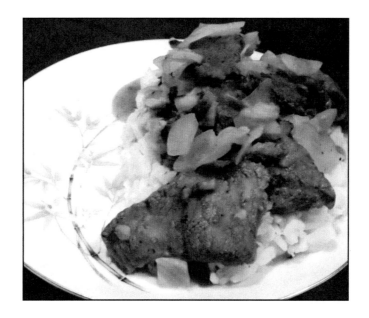

Beef Stir Fry

Prep Time: 20 min.

Cook Time: 20 min.

Makes: 4-6 servings

2 Tbsp canola oil

2 c cabbage, chopped

1 c yellow or green onions, diced

1 c mushrooms, sliced

1 c cubed beef steak

1 Tbsp brown sugar

1 Tbsp rice vinegar

2 c cold water mixed with 2 Tbsp cornstarch

salt and pepper to taste

cooked white rice to plate

1. In large skillet, add canola oil, cabbage, onions, and mushrooms. Cook on medium heat and cover.

2. Add meat to skillet, along with brown sugar and rice vinegar. Stir and keep covered until cabbage softens and beef browns.

3. When close to done, pour cornstarch mixture into skillet. Add salt and pepper. Stir to keep from sticking until it thickens. Serve over cooked rice.

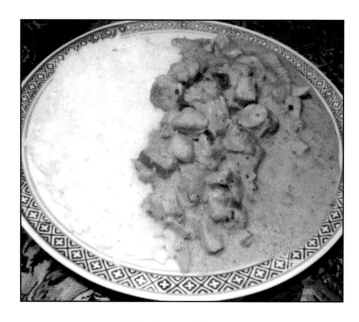

Chicken Curry

Prep Time: 15 min.

Cook Time: 20 min.

Makes: 4 servings

1 Tbsp canola oil

2 c chicken breast, cubed

1/2 c onions, chopped

1/2 tsp salt

1/4 tsp pepper

1 Tbsp curry powder

1 tsp sugar

1/2 tsp crushed red pepper

1 c cream mixed with 1 tsp cornstarch

cooked rice to plate

1. Heat oil in deep pan on stove. Add chicken pieces and onions, fry until white.

2. Sprinkle on salt, pepper, curry powder, sugar, and red pepper. Cook until sauce starts to thicken and chicken is coated. Add cream mixture, cook until set. Serve over rice.

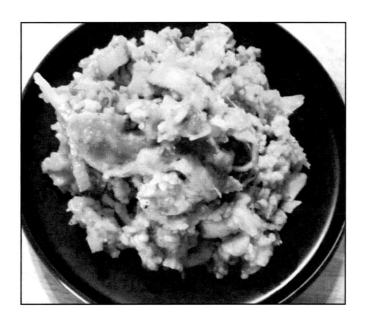

Bacon Chicken Curry

Prep Time: 15 min.
Cook Time: 20-25 min.
Makes: 4-6 servings

1/2 cabbage, cut thin
2 stalks celery, diced
2 Tbsp olive oil
1 piece chicken breast, cubed
4 pieces of bacon
4 green onion sprigs, chopped
1 tsp curry powder
1/2 c brown sugar
1 tsp pepper
1/4 c cornstarch mixed with 1 c cold water
2 Tbsp chicken base
1 tsp balsamic vinegar
cooked white rice

1. In skillet, fry cabbage and celery in olive oil. Add chicken pieces, bacon, and green onions. When chicken is cooked, add curry powder, brown sugar, pepper, cornstarch mix, chicken base, and balsamic vinegar. Stir well.

2. Cook until sauce forms around vegetables, stirring to keep it from burning. Serve over rice.

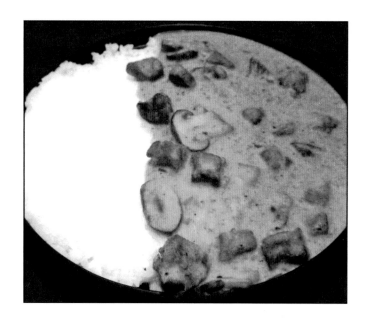

Beef Curry

Prep Time: 15 min.
Cook Time: 20 min.
Makes: 4-6 servings

1 Tbsp butter

2 c beef, cubed

1/4 tsp salt

1/4 tsp pepper

1 c mushrooms, sliced

1 Tbsp curry powder

1 tsp sugar

1 tsp brown sugar

1/2 tsp crushed red pepper

2 c cold beef broth mixed with 2 Tbsp cornstarch

1/2 c green onions, chopped

1 c cream

cooked rice to plate

1. Heat butter in a deep pan on the stove. Add beef cubes, salt, pepper, and mushrooms. Cover and fry until browned.

2. Sprinkle on curry powder, sugar, brown sugar, and red pepper.

3. Add beef broth mix and green onions. Cover and cook until sauce starts to thicken. Add cream, uncover and cook until set. Serve over rice.

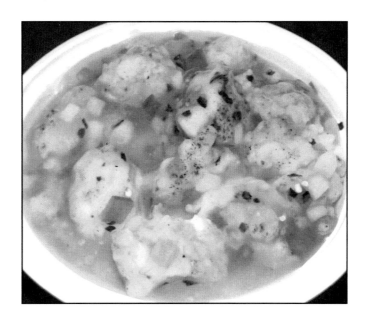

General Tso's Chicken

Prep Time: 20 min.
Cook Time: 25-30 min.
Makes: 4-6 servings

1 c cornstarch (divided)
1 tsp onion flakes
1/4 c sugar
2 Tbsp mirin
1/8 c white vinegar
2 Tbsp chicken base mixed with 2 c water
2 eggs, beaten
1 tsp seasoning salt
1 tsp salt
1 tsp pepper
2 lbs chicken breast, cubed
1/4 c oil
2 c green onions
1 tsp crushed red pepper

1. In bowl, make a sauce by mixing together 1/4 c cornstarch, onion flakes, sugar, mirin, vinegar, and chicken base mixture. Set aside.

2. In bowl, mix egg, seasoning salt, salt, pepper, and remaining cornstarch. Coat chicken pieces, fry in hot oil until crispy. Drain on paper towel.

3. In saucepan, stir fry green onions and crushed red pepper for 1 min. Add sauce and chicken pieces, cooking until warmed (1-2 min).

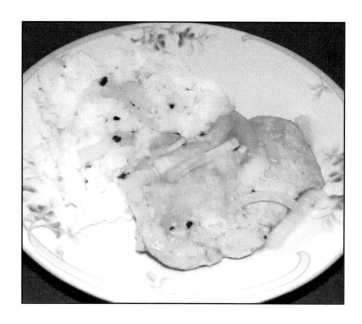

Asian Glazed Pork Chops

Prep Time: 5 min.

Cook Time: 20 min.

Makes: 2 servings

2 Tbsp olive oil

2 pork chops

1 Tbsp brown sugar

1 tsp salt

2 Tbsp rice vinegar

1 tsp cornstarch

1/4 tsp crushed red pepper (optional)

1/2 c onion slices

cooked white rice to plate

1. In skillet, heat olive oil. Brown chops on one side. In bowl, whisk together brown sugar, salt, rice vinegar, cornstarch, and crushed red pepper. Set aside.

2. Turn chops and add onion slices. Whisk in sauce. Simmer until pork chops cook through and sauce has thickened. Serve with white rice.

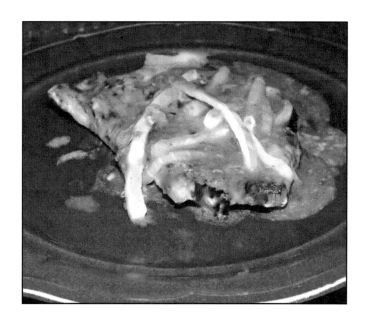

Asian Glazed Beef Steaks

Prep Time: 5 min.

Cook Time: 20 min.

Makes: 2 servings

2 Tbsp olive oil

2 beef steaks

1 Tbsp brown sugar

1 tsp salt

2 Tbsp rice vinegar

1 tsp cornstarch

1/4 tsp crushed red pepper (optional)

1/2 c onion slices

cooked white rice to plate

1. In skillet, heat olive oil. Brown steaks on one side. In bowl, whisk together brown sugar, salt, rice vinegar, cornstarch, and crushed red pepper. Set aside.

2. Turn steaks and add onion slices. Whisk in sauce. Simmer until beef steaks have cooked through and sauce has thickened. Serve with white rice.

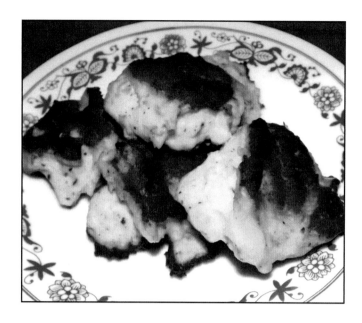

Meatballs

Prep Time: 10 min.

Cook Time: 15-20 min.

Makes: 2-3 servings

2 chicken breasts, diced

1 egg

2 green onions

1 tsp chicken base

salt and pepper to taste

1/4 tsp red wine vinegar

1 tsp Italian seasoning

1 tsp onion powder

2 tsp all-purpose rice flour blend

1/4 c olive oil

1. Blend together chicken, egg, green onions, chicken base, salt, pepper, red wine vinegar, Italian seasoning, onion powder, and rice flour in food processor until smooth.

2. Heat oil in pan. Drop mixture by spoon and cook until browned. Serve over spaghetti or with sauce.

Variations: Can use beef or pork pieces for chicken.

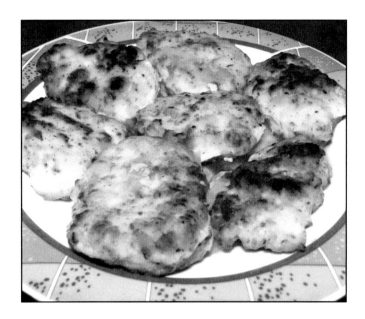

Sweet and Sour Meatballs

Prep Time: 20 min.
Cook Time: 20 min.
Makes: 2-3 servings

Meatball Ingredients:

1 tsp onion powder	2 chicken breasts, diced
1 egg	2 green onions
1 tsp chicken base	pepper to taste
1/4 tsp red wine vinegar	1 tsp Italian seasoning
2 tsp all-purpose rice flour blend	

Sauce Ingredients:

1/2 c honey

1 Tbsp onion flakes

1/2 tsp salt

1 Tbsp mirin

2 tsp onion powder

1 c cold water mixed with 1 Tbsp cornstarch

For the skillet:

1/2 c olive oil or canola oil

1. Blend together meatball ingredients in food processor until smooth.

2. Heat oil on medium-low heat in skillet. Drop meat blend by spoonful into pan. Brown on one side, flip and cook through.

3. In saucepan, combine honey, onion flakes, salt, mirin, cornstarch mixture, and vinegar. Stir and cook over medium heat until it thickens. Dip cooked meatballs into sauce and serve.

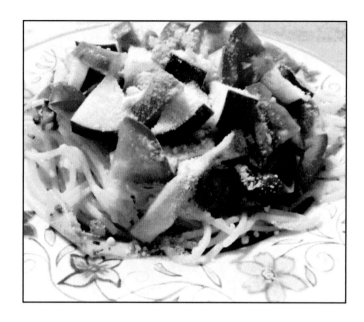

Tomato Cucumber Spaghetti

Prep Time: 15 min.

Cook Time: 25 min.

Makes: 2 servings

1/2 lb corn spaghetti noodles

1 piece chicken breast, cubed

4 large mushrooms, sliced

1 sprig green onions, diced

1 Tbsp butter

2 Tbsp oregano or Italian seasoning

1/4 cucumber, diced

1/2 Roma tomato, diced

parmesan cheese to taste

1. Cook spaghetti in pot until cooked, but firm. Drain and rinse thoroughly.

2. In saucepan, cook chicken, mushrooms, and green onions in butter. Add oregano, cook until warm. Spread over noodles. Top with cucumber, tomato, and parmesan cheese on serving to be eaten.

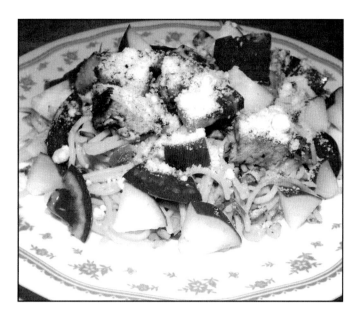

Corn Spaghetti

Prep Time: 15 min.

Cook Time: 30 min.

Makes: 2 servings

1/2 lb corn spaghetti noodles

1 piece boneless, skinless chicken breast

2 Tbsp dry ranch dressing mix (p.2)

4 large mushrooms, sliced

1 sprig green onions, diced

1 c corn

1 Tbsp butter

2 Tbsp oregano or Italian seasoning

1/4 cucumber, diced

1/2 Roma tomato, diced

parmesan cheese to taste

1. Cook spaghetti in pot until cooked, but firm. Drain and rinse thoroughly.

2. In saucepan, add chicken and sprinkle with ranch dressing mix. Cook and slice into pieces; set aside.

3. Sauté mushrooms, green onions, and corn in butter. Add oregano and chicken pieces. Cook until warm. Spread over noodles. Top with cucumber, tomato, and parmesan on serving to be eaten.

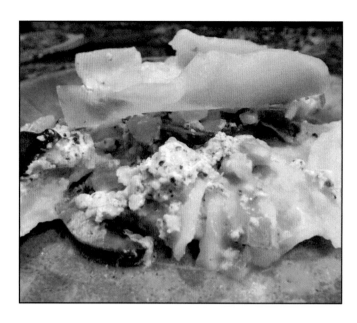

Slow Cooker Lasagna

Prep Time: 20 min.
Cook Time: 2 hrs.
Makes: 4 servings

1 c cottage cheese
1 pkg (8 oz) cream cheese, softened
1/2 c sour cream
1 Tbsp Italian seasoning
2 c chicken breast, cubed
1 c mushrooms, sliced
1 c onions, chopped
1 box oven ready corn lasagna noodles
2 c shredded white cheese
1/4 c water

1. In bowl, combine cottage cheese, cream cheese, sour cream, and Italian seasoning to make a sauce. In greased slow cooker, add 2/3 c chicken, a layer of sauce, 1/3 c mushrooms, 1/3 c onions, 3 lasagna noodles, and 2/3 c cheese.

2. Repeat twice more, adding cheese on the top. Pour water, cook on high 2 hrs. until noodles are soft.

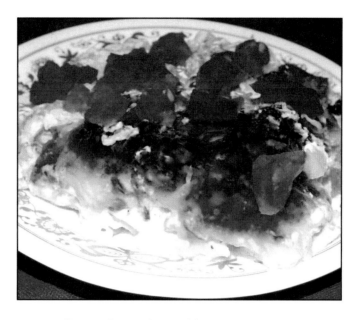

Oven Baked Beef Roast Lasagna

Prep Time: 20 min.

Cook Time: 1 hr.

Makes: 2 pans

2 pkgs cream cheese, softened   1/4 c milk

1 Tbsp Italian seasoning   1 c sour cream

1 tsp salt   1/4 c parmesan cheese

2 onions, chopped   2 green onions, diced

2 c beef roast, shredded   1/2 cabbage, diced

4 c shredded cheddar cheese   4 c shredded mozzarella cheese

2 pkgs corn lasagna noodles   1 c water

4 Roma tomatoes, diced

1. Preheat oven to 400°F. In bowl, mix cream cheese, milk, Italian seasoning, sour cream, salt, and parmesan until blended. Sauté onions.

2. In bowl, combine green onions, beef roast, cabbage, and sautéed onions. In separate bowl, stir together cheeses. Layer in greased baking dish: lasagna noodles, cream cheese spread, meat and veggies, and cheese, alternating until filled. Add 1 c water to pan.

3. Cover with tin foil and bake 1 hr. Top with diced tomatoes on portion to be eaten.

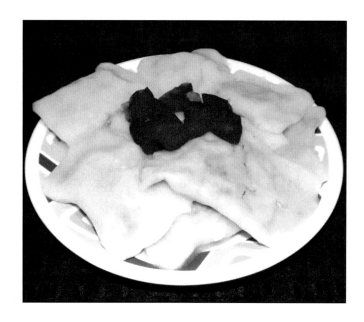

Raviolis

Prep Time: 2 hrs.
Cook Time: 10-15 min.
Makes: 40-50 raviolis

1 c beef, pork, or chicken, cubed
1/3 c minced onion
1 egg
2 Tbsp parmesan cheese
1 Tbsp Italian seasoning
1/2 tsp salt
1 ball all-purpose rice flour dough (p.182)
1/2 c water
2 Tbsp olive oil

1. In skillet, cook beef cubes and onions. Chop meat and onions in food processor.

2. In medium bowl, stir together meat, egg, parmesan cheese, Italian seasoning, and salt until mixed well.

3. Roll out dough on floured surface. Cut out small rectangles. In middle of each rectangle, spoon some meat mixture, then fold over and seal dough. Cook in skillet with water and oil until cooked through, about 10-15 min. Serve with diced tomato on top or cheese sauce if desired.

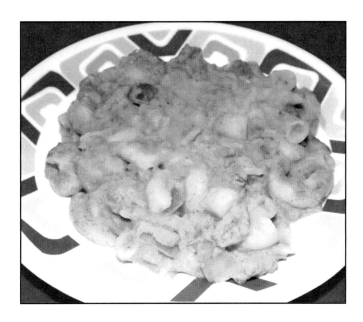

Beef Stroganoff

Prep Time: 20 min.
Cook Time: 20 min.
Makes: 4-6 servings

3/4 c onions, chopped

2 Tbsp butter

2 c cooked roast, cubed

1 tsp onion powder

1/2 tsp salt

1/2 tsp pepper

1 pkg (8 oz) chopped fresh mushrooms

1 c cooked corn noodles

1 Tbsp cornstarch

1 c cold beef broth (p.185)

1 c sour cream

1. In skillet, sauté onions in butter until tender. Add roast, onion powder, salt, pepper, mushrooms, and noodles. Stir and cook until heated.

2. In cup, combine cornstarch and beef broth. Pour into skillet with the sour cream. Stir and cook until thickened. Eat warm.

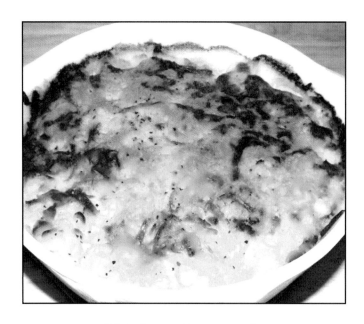

Chicken Casserole

Prep Time: 20 min.

Cook Time: 45 min.

Makes: 4 servings

1 c cold chicken broth (p.184)

1 Tbsp cornstarch

2 c chicken, cubed

1/2 c cooked bacon pieces, crumbled

2 c cooked corn pasta

salt and pepper to taste

1 c shredded Colby Jack cheese

1. Preheat oven to 400°F. In saucepan, combine broth and cornstarch. Whisk on medium heat until thickened.

2. In bowl, combine chicken, bacon, pasta, and sauce. Stir until incorporated.

3. Pour into greased 9x9 pan or casserole dish. Sprinkle top with salt, pepper, and shredded cheese. Bake for 45 min. or until chicken is cooked through.

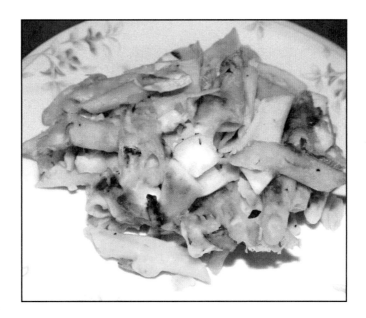

Veggie Pasta Casserole

Prep Time: 10 min.

Cook Time: 30 min.

Makes: 4 servings

1/2 c onions, chopped

1 c zucchini, chopped

1 c yellow summer squash, chopped

2 c cooked corn penne pasta

2 Tbsp olive oil

salt and pepper to taste

1 c water

1 c shredded cheese

1. Preheat oven to 375°F. In skillet, sauté onions until golden. In medium bowl, add onions, zucchini, summer squash, and pasta. Coat with olive oil. Sprinkle on salt and pepper.

2. Pour vegetables into greased 9x9 baking dish or casserole dish. Add water. Cook 20 min. Top with shredded cheese, cook 10 more min. until cheese is melted and veggies are softened. Serve hot.

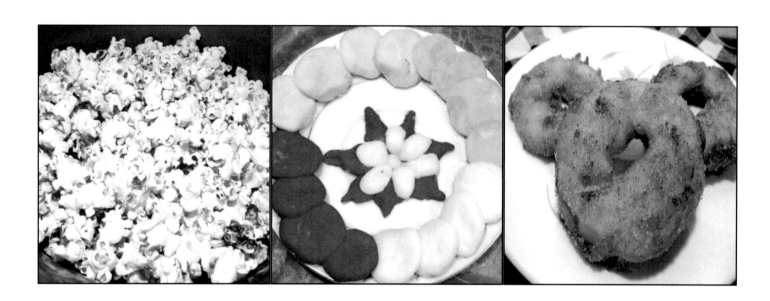

Desserts and Breads

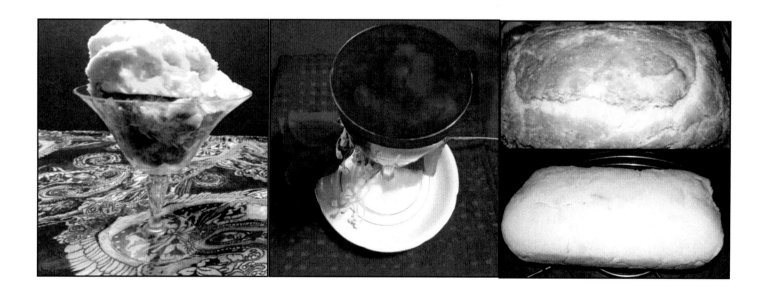

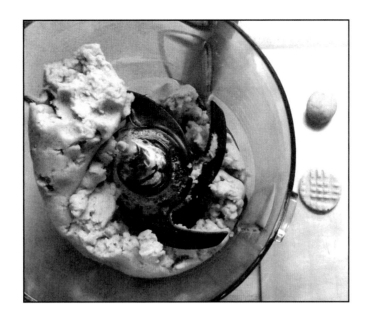

Brown Sugar Pastry

Prep Time: 5 min.
Cook Time: 10 min. per tray
Makes: 3-4 dozen cookies

1 c all-purpose rice flour blend

1/2 c brown sugar

1/2 c butter, salted

1/2 tsp cinnamon

1 large egg

1. In dough mixer or in bowl, mix together rice flour, brown sugar, butter, cinnamon, and egg until it forms a dough.

2. For cookies, preheat oven to 350°F. Roll dough into balls and flatten with a fork. Bake for 10 min. until cookies are golden. Cool 2 minutes and remove from tray. Cookies should be crumbly.

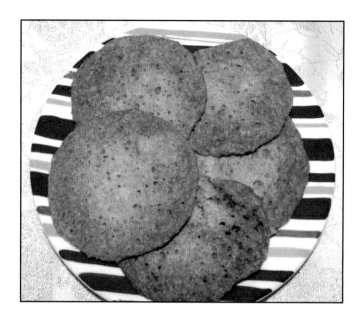

Lace Cookies

Prep Time: 15 min.
Cook Time: 10 min. per tray
Makes: 4-5 dozen cookies

2/3 c butter or lard, softened

1 1/2 c sugar

2 eggs

1 tsp vanilla

1 tsp vinegar

1 2/3 c all-purpose rice flour blend

1 tsp baking soda

1 tsp salt

1 tsp cinnamon

1. Preheat oven to 350°F. In bowl, cream butter and 1 c sugar. Beat in eggs, vanilla, and vinegar. In separate bowl, sift flour, soda, and salt together.

2. Blend dry ingredients into egg mixture. Add remaining sugar and cinnamon; stir. Drop cookie dough from teaspoon onto cookie sheet, 2-in. apart. Bake 10 min. or until browned and spread flat. Cool 1 min. and remove quickly from tray.

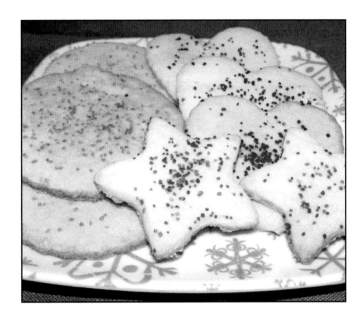

Sugar Cookies

Prep Time: 15 min.
Cook Time: 7-9 min.
Makes: 2-3 dozen

1 1/2 c all-purpose rice flour blend

1 tsp baking soda

1/2 c sugar

1/2 tsp salt

1/2 c butter

1/2 tsp vinegar

1 tsp vanilla extract

1/4 c sour cream

1/4 c milk or cream

colored sugar or sprinkles for top

1. Preheat oven to 375°F. In bowl, combine rice flour, baking soda, sugar, and salt. Cut in butter until crumbly.

2. Stir in vinegar, vanilla, sour cream, and milk; stir. Turn on floured surface and roll out. Cut into desired shapes. Top each cookie with sugar.

3. Place on cookie sheet. Bake 7-9 min. until lightly browned.

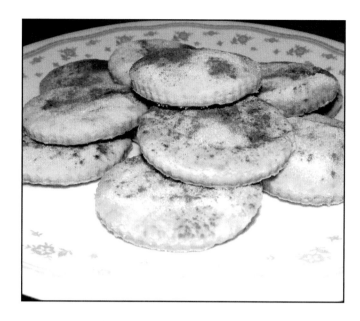

Cinnamon Cookies

Prep Time: 15 min.
Cook Time: 7-9 min.
Makes: 2-3 dozen

1 1/2 c all-purpose rice flour blend

1/2 tsp baking soda

1/2 c sugar

1/2 tsp salt

1/2 c butter

1/2 tsp vinegar

1 tsp vanilla extract

1/4 c sour cream

1 tsp cinnamon

1/4 c milk

cinnamon sugar for top (optional)

1. Preheat oven to 400°F. In bowl, combine flour, baking soda, sugar, and salt. Cut in butter until crumbly. Stir in vinegar, vanilla, sour cream, cinnamon, and milk.

2. Turn dough on floured surface and roll out. Cut into desired shapes. Place on cookie sheet.

3. Bake 7-9 min. or until lightly browned. Sprinkle with cinnamon sugar.

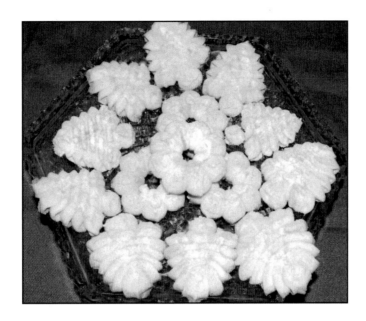

Spritz Cookies
Prep Time: 15 min.
Cook Time: 8-9 min.
Makes: 3-4 dozen cookies

3/4 c butter, softened

1/2 c sugar

1 egg

1 tsp vanilla OR 1/2 tsp vanilla and 1/2 tsp flavoring (mint, rum, cherry, etc.)

2 c all-purpose rice flour blend

1. Preheat oven to 400°F. In medium bowl, cream butter and sugar together. Beat in egg and vanilla.

2. Sift in rice flour, 1/4 at a time, mixing well to make a dough. Spoon into spritzer or pastry tube. Choose desired shape nozzle and press onto ungreased cookie sheet. Bake 8-9 min. or until lightly browned. Cool and serve.

Variations: Can add food coloring or sprinkles to make colorful.

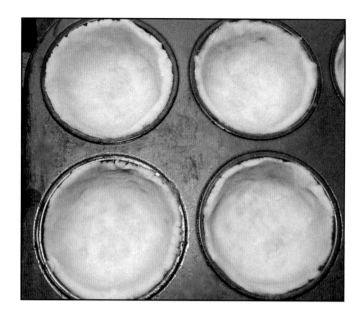

Rice Flour Pie Crust

Prep Time: 20 min.

Makes: 8 mini pies or 1 9-in. pie

1 large egg, beaten

1/4 c melted butter

1 c rice flour or all-purpose rice flour blend

1 Tbsp sugar

1 dash salt

1. In medium bowl, beat egg and butter together. Add rice flour, sugar, and salt. Mix until it forms a dough, adding rice flour and water as needed to form the right consistency.

2. Shape dough to fit greased pie pan or muffin tins for mini pies. Can also freeze dough until needed.

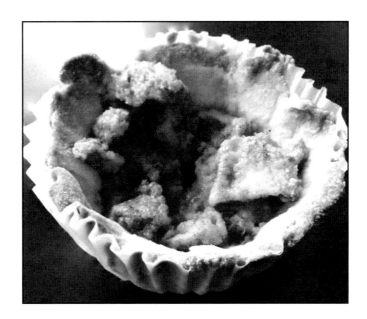

Mini Apple Pies

Prep Time: 20 min.

Cook Time: 25-30 min.

Makes: 6 mini pies

2 c apples, cored, sliced, and peeled

2 Tbsp white sugar

1/2 tsp cinnamon

dash salt

2 Tbsp all-purpose rice flour blend

rice flour pie crust (p.136)

2 Tbsp butter, cubed

1. Preheat oven to 350°F. In bowl, combine apples, sugar, cinnamon, salt, and rice flour. Stir until apples are coated. Press dough into greased muffin tins.

2. Spoon pie filling into each tin. Add cubed butter to the top of each. Cook for 25-30 min. or until golden brown.

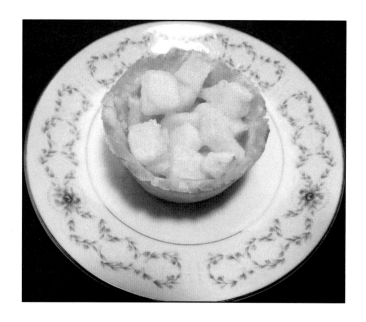

Mini Pear Pies

Prep Time: 20 min.

Cook Time: 25-30 min.

Makes: 6 mini pies

2 c pears, cored, cubed, and peeled

2 Tbsp white sugar

dash salt

2 Tbsp all-purpose rice flour blend

rice flour pie crust (p.136)

2 Tbsp butter, cubed

1. Preheat oven to 350°F. In bowl, combine pears, sugar, salt, and rice flour. Stir until pears are coated. Press dough into greased muffin tins.

2. Spoon pie filling into each tin. Add cubed butter to the top of each. Cook for 25-30 min. or until golden brown.

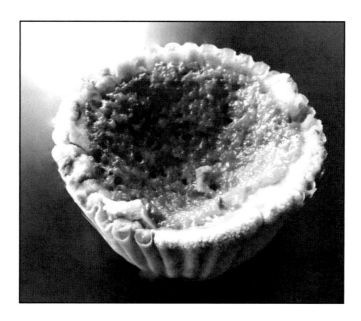

Mini Syrup Pies

Prep Time: 20 min.

Cook Time: 25-30 min.

Makes: 4-6 mini pies

rice flour pie crust (p.136)

1 Tbsp melted butter

1 egg, beaten

1/3 c sugar

dash salt

1/3 c dark corn syrup

1. Preheat oven to 350°F. Press dough into greased muffin tin. In bowl, add melted butter to beaten egg; stir.

2. Add sugar, salt, and corn syrup to egg mixture. Mix well. Pour into mini pie crusts 3/4 full. Cook for 25-30 min. or until lightly browned.

Variations: If using light corn syrup, use brown sugar.

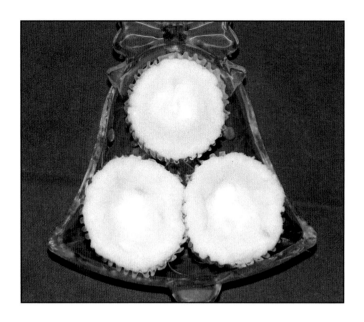

Mini Cheesecake Tarts

Prep Time: 25 min.

Cook Time: 20-25 min.

Makes: 12 - 18 cheesecake tarts

rice flour pie crust (p.136)

2 pkgs (8 oz each) cream cheese, softened

2/3 c sugar

2 eggs

2 tsp vanilla extract

1. Preheat oven to 325°F. Roll out dough on floured surface and cut into circles. In cupcake-lined muffin tins, insert a circle of dough in each tin.

2. In bowl, beat cream cheese and sugar with egg beater on medium speed until light and fluffy. Add eggs and vanilla; beat well.

3. Spoon batter into each muffin tin. Bake 20-25 min. or until set. Remove from pans and cool. Top with favorite toppings.

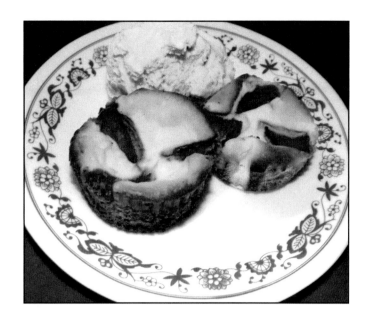

Strawberry Cheesecake Tarts

Prep Time: 25 min.

Cook Time: 40-45 min.

Makes: 12 - 18 mini tarts

rice flour pie crust (p.136)

1 1/2 pkgs (12 oz) cream cheese, softened

1/2 c butter, softened

2 eggs

1/2 c sugar

1 tsp vanilla

1 c sliced strawberries

1. Preheat oven to 375°F. Roll out dough on floured surface and cut into circles. In cupcake-lined muffin tins, insert a circle of dough into each tin.

2. Microwave cream cheese and butter for 1 min. Add eggs, sugar, and vanilla. Stir until smooth. Spoon in cream cheese mixture into tins, 2/3 full.

3. Add strawberry slices to center of each tart. Cook 40-45 min. or until tops are golden and set.

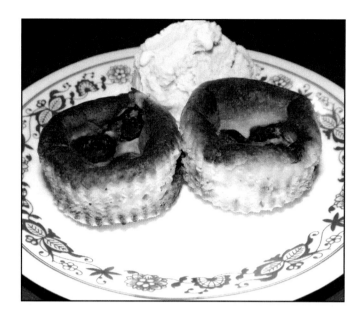

Blueberry Cheesecake Tarts

Prep Time: 25 min.

Cook Time: 40-45 min.

Makes: 12 - 18 mini tarts

rice flour pie crust (p.136)

1 1/2 pkgs (12 oz) cream cheese, softened

1/2 c butter, softened

2 eggs

1/2 c sugar

1 tsp vanilla

1/2 c blueberries

1. Preheat oven to 375°F. Roll out dough on floured surface and cut into circles. In cupcake-lined muffin tins, insert a circle of dough into each tin.

2. Microwave cream cheese and butter for 1 min. Add eggs, sugar, and vanilla. Stir until smooth. Spoon in cream cheese mixture into tins, 2/3 full.

3. Add blueberries to center of each tart. Cook 40-45 min. or until tops are golden and set.

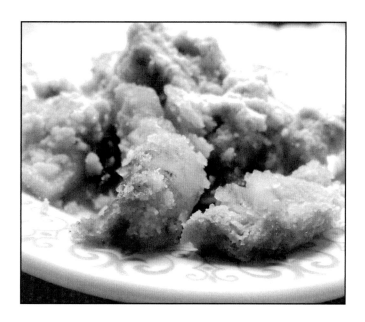

Apple Crisp

Prep Time: 20 min.

Cook Time: 40 min.

Makes: 1 pan

3 to 4 apples, cored, peeled, and sliced

2 Tbsp all-purpose rice flour blend

1 Tbsp butter

1/2 c brown sugar

1/2 tsp cinnamon

brown sugar pastry dough (p.131)

1. Preheat oven to 350°F. In medium bowl, combine apples, rice flour, butter, brown sugar, and cinnamon until apples are coated.

2. In greased 9x9 baking pan, pour apple mixture in, then carefully top it with the brown sugar pastry dough. Press in and bake for 40 min. It should come out a little grainy.

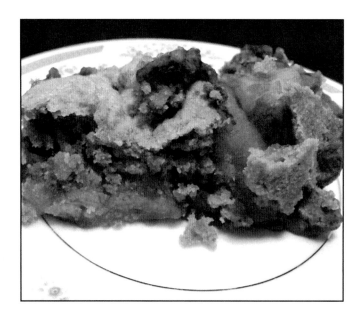

Pear Crisp

Prep Time: 20 min.

Cook Time: 40 min.

Makes: 1 pan

3 to 4 pears, cored, peeled, and sliced

2 Tbsp all-purpose rice flour blend

1 Tbsp butter

1/2 c brown sugar

1/2 tsp cinnamon

brown sugar pastry dough (p.131)

1. Preheat oven to 350°F. In medium bowl, combine pears, rice flour, butter, brown sugar, and cinnamon until pears are coated.

2. In greased 9x9 baking pan, pour pear mixture in, then carefully top it with the brown sugar pastry dough. Press in and bake for 40 min. It should come out a little grainy.

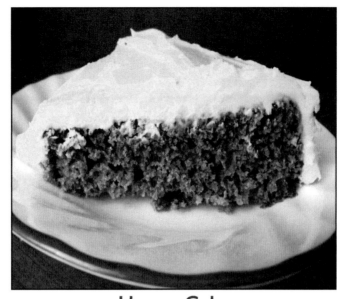

Honey Cake

Prep Time: 10-15 min.

Cook Time: 30 min.

Makes: 10-12 servings

1/4 c lard

1/2 c sugar

1/4 c honey

1 tsp vanilla

1 egg

1/2 tsp salt

1 tsp baking soda

1 c all-purpose rice flour blend

1/4 c buttermilk

1. Preheat oven to 350°F. In bowl, cream lard and sugar. Add honey, vanilla, and egg. Mix well.

2. Add rice flour, salt, and soda, mixing in. Add buttermilk, mix. Pour in greased 8x8, 9x9, or round cake pan. Bake 30 min. or until toothpick comes out clean. Eat plain or top with frosting.

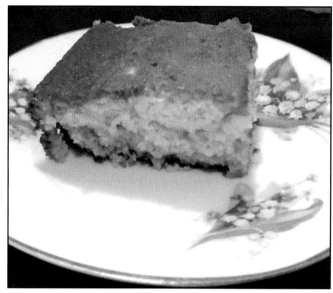

Hot Milk Sponge Cake

Prep Time: 20 min.

Cook Time: 25 min.

Makes: 1 cake

1 c white sugar

2 eggs

1 c all-purpose rice flour blend

1 tsp baking soda

1 tsp vinegar

2 Tbsp butter, melted

1/2 c hot milk

1 tsp vanilla

1. Preheat oven to 350°F. In bowl, combine white sugar and eggs. Beat well. Add rice flour, baking soda, and vinegar. Set aside.

2. In bowl, mix melted butter with hot milk. Combine with rice flour mixture. Add vanilla, stir until incorporated. Pour in 9x9 greased baking pan. Bake 20 min. or until cooked through.

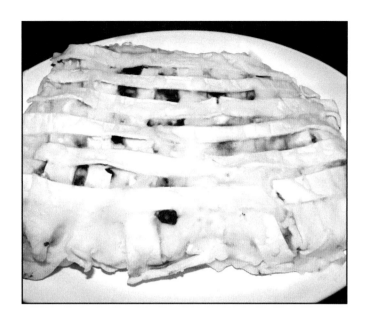

Cherry Cheese Strudel

Prep Time: 30 min.
Cook Time: 25-30 min.
Makes: 12 servings

1 pkg (8 oz) cream cheese, softened
1/3 c powdered sugar
1 egg, separated
1/2 tsp vanilla extract
1 ball all-purpose rice flour dough (p.182)
1 c fresh or thawed frozen pitted cherries
Glaze: 1/2 c powdered sugar
1 Tbsp milk

1. Preheat oven to 375°F. In bowl, combine cream cheese, powdered sugar, egg yolk, and vanilla until smooth. Spread out 1/2 dough onto greased baking sheet, making a rectangle.

2. Spread cream cheese mix over dough 1/2-in. from edge. Top with cherries. On floured surface, roll out remaining dough and cut into strips. Place on top of cherries and seal outer edges to bottom of dough. Brush strips with beaten egg wash.

3. Bake 25-30 min. until golden brown. For glaze, stir powdered sugar with milk until smooth. Drizzle.

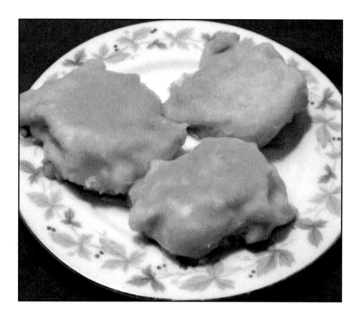

Maple Bars
Prep Time: 15 min.
Cook Time: 15 min.
Makes: 1 dozen bars

1/4 c butter

1/2 c brown sugar

3 Tbsp milk

1 Tbsp corn syrup

2 tsp pancake syrup

2 c powdered sugar

fried Chinese donuts (p.156)

1. In saucepan, combine butter and brown sugar. Whisk in milk and heat on medium heat for 5 min., stirring constantly. Melt butter and dissolve sugar, remove from heat.

2. Add corn syrup and pancake syrup; stir. Add powdered sugar, 1/2 c at a time, stirring until smooth each time. Add more milk if necessary. Keep warm on the stove, stirring occasionally.

3. Dip each donut in the glaze mixture. Let cool on rack.

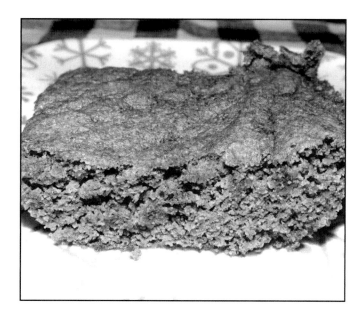

Spice Bars

Prep Time: 15 min.
Cook Time: 20-25 min.
Makes: 9-12 servings

1/2 c butter, softened

1/2 c sugar

1/2 c packed brown sugar

1 egg

1 tsp vanilla

1/4 c molasses

1 tsp cinnamon

1/2 tsp salt

1/8 tsp nutmeg

1 tsp baking soda

2 c all-purpose rice flour blend

1/2 c buttermilk OR milk + 1 Tbsp vinegar

1. Preheat oven to 350°F. Mix butter and sugars together until fluffy. Add egg, vanilla, and molasses. Beat until light brown. Add cinnamon, salt, nutmeg, and baking soda; stir.

2. Sift in 1 c rice flour and stir until smooth. Add buttermilk and stir. Add the rest of the rice flour, stir until incorporated. Do not over mix.

3. Pour into greased 9x9 or 9x13 pan. Bake 20-25 min. until a toothpick in center comes out clean.

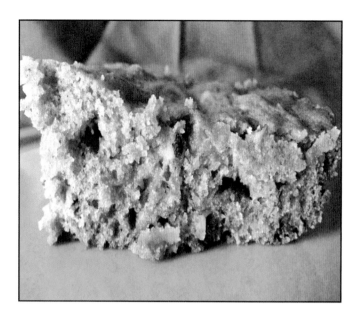

Zucchini Bars

Prep Time: 15 min.
Cook Time: 35 min.
Makes: 12 servings

3/4 c butter, softened

1/2 c brown sugar

1/2 c white sugar

2 eggs

1 tsp vanilla

1 3/4 c all-purpose rice flour blend

1 tsp baking soda

1/2 tsp salt

1 tsp cinnamon

2 c zucchini, peeled and shredded

1. Preheat oven to 350°F. In bowl, cream together butter, sugars, and eggs until smooth.

2. Add in vanilla, rice flour, soda, salt, cinnamon, and zucchini. Mix well. Bake in a greased 9x13 pan for 35 min. Cool and serve with whip topping or frosting.

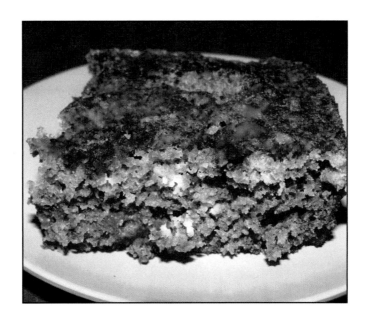

Strawberry Rhubarb Bars

Prep Time: 10 min.
Cook Time: 30 min.
Makes: 12 servings

3 Tbsp butter
1/2 c sugar
1 egg
1/2 tsp salt
1 tsp baking soda
3/4 c all-purpose rice flour blend
1 tsp vanilla
1 c strawberry-rhubarb jam (p.189)

1. Preheat oven to 350°F. In bowl, cream butter and sugar together. Add egg; mix. Add salt, soda, and rice flour. Mix well.

2. Add vanilla and strawberry-rhubarb jam. Mix just until incorporated, being careful not to over mix. Pour in a greased 9x9 cake pan.

3. Bake 30 min. until toothpick comes out clean and is springy to the touch in the middle. Cool and eat plain or top with powdered sugar, whip topping, or butter cream frosting.

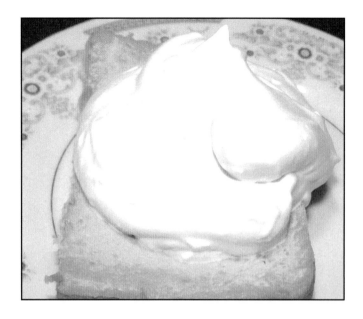

Berry Custard

Prep Time: 20 min.

Cook Time: 30 min.

Makes: 9-12 servings

3/4 c (6 oz) cream cheese, softened

2/3 c plain yogurt

1 Tbsp all-purpose rice flour blend

2 Tbsp sugar

1/4 tsp salt

4 egg whites

1/2 c choice of berries (fresh or thawed frozen)

1. Preheat oven to 350°F. Using blender, mix together cream cheese, yogurt, rice flour, sugar, salt, egg whites, and fruit until blended.

2. In greased 9x9 pan, pour in batter. Cook 30 min. or until set and cooked through. Top with whip cream or ice cream.

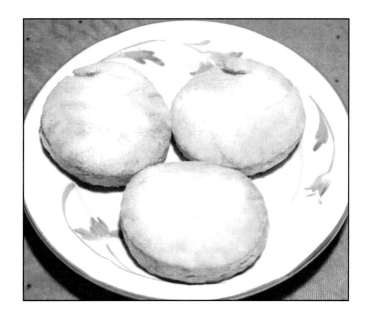

Easy Scones

Prep Time: 20 min.
Cook Time: 12-15 min.
Makes: 18-24 scones

1 1/2 c all-purpose rice flour blend

1/4 c sugar

1/2 tsp salt

1/2 c cold butter

1/2 tsp baking soda

1/2 tsp vinegar

1 tsp vanilla extract

1/4 c sour cream or plain yogurt

1/4 c buttermilk

sugar for tops (optional)

1. Preheat oven to 400°F. In bowl, combine flour, sugar, and salt. Cut in butter until crumbly. Stir in baking soda, vinegar, vanilla, sour cream, and buttermilk.

2. Turn dough on floured surface, pressing 1/2-in. thick. Cut into 3-in. round circles. Place on greased cookie sheet. Sugar tops of each scone if desired.

3. Bake 12-15 min. or until lightly browned.

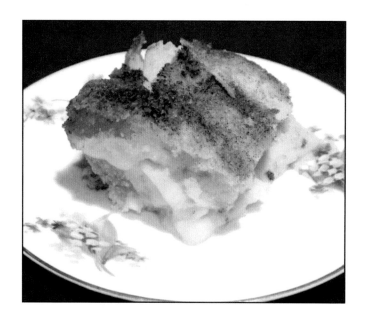

Cheesecake Scones

Prep Time: 25 min.

Cook Time: 20-30 min.

Makes: 1 pan

2 pkg (8 oz each) cream cheese, softened

1 c sugar

1 1/2 tsp vanilla

easy scones dough (p.153)

1/4 c butter, melted

1 tsp cinnamon mixed with 2 Tbsp sugar

1. Preheat oven to 350°F. In bowl, combine cream cheese, sugar, and vanilla until smooth.

Press in 1/2 scone dough in greased 9x9 pan. Spread cream cheese mix over dough.

2. Drizzle butter over cream cheese. Layer remaining dough over cream cheese spread.

Sprinkle with cinnamon sugar mix.

3. Bake 20-30 min. or until golden.

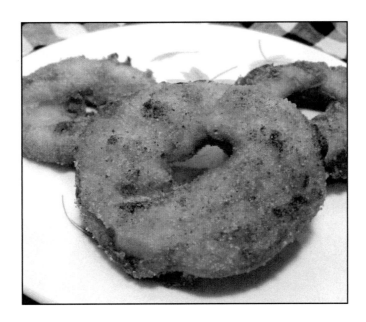

Fried Cinnamon Apple Rings

Prep Time: 20 min.
Cook Time: 20-25 min.
Makes: 3-4 dozen apple rings

1 c all-purpose rice flour blend

1/4 tsp baking soda

2 Tbsp sugar

1/4 tsp salt

1/8 tsp cinnamon

1 large egg, beaten

1/4 tsp vinegar

1 c buttermilk

Topping: 1 c sugar mixed with 2 Tbsp cinnamon

4 large apples, peeled

canola oil for pan

1. In large bowl, combine rice flour, baking soda, sugar, salt, and cinnamon. Set aside. In a small bowl, combine egg, vinegar, and buttermilk.

2. In third bowl, set aside cinnamon sugar topping. Slice apples into 1/4-in. thick circles, discarding the core pieces.

3. Heat oil in a pan. Combine rice flour mixture with buttermilk mixture, creating a batter. Dip each apple ring in batter, fry until golden crispy, dab with paper towel, and coat with cinnamon sugar. Serve warm.

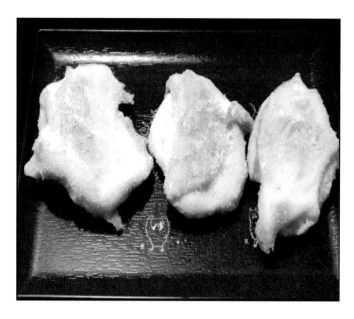

Fried Chinese Donuts

Prep Time: 15 min.

Cook Time: about 20 min.

Makes: 12 donuts

1 1/2 c all-purpose rice flour blend

1 c milk

1 egg

1 Tbsp melted butter

1 Tbsp sugar

1 tsp vanilla extract

1/2 c canola oil, for frying

sugar to top

1. Preheat oven to 350°F. In bowl, combine rice flour, milk, egg, melted butter, sugar, and vanilla until blended.

2. Heat canola oil in skillet. When oil is hot, drop batter in by spoonful. Brown on both sides.

3. Place on cookie sheet and bake 8 min. until centers are cooked. Sprinkle with sugar and cool. Can be eaten plain or topped with fruit or ice cream.

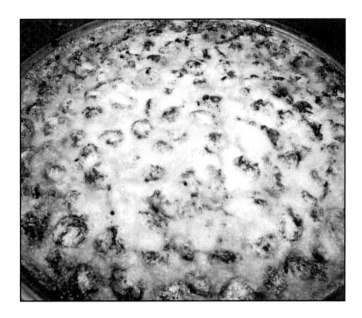

Cherry Dessert

Prep Time: 25 min.

Cook Time: 40-50 min.

Makes: 8 servings

2 Tbsp and 1 c sugar, divided

2 1/2 c cherries, pitted

4 eggs

1/4 tsp salt

3/4 c all-purpose rice flour blend

1 tsp vanilla

1 c milk

2 Tbsp melted butter

1. Preheat oven to 350°F. Grease a 10-in. round cake pan or pie pan. Dust with 2 Tbsp sugar and layer in cherries. In mixing bowl, add eggs, remaining sugar, and salt; whisk together.

2. Add rice flour until incorporated. Stir in vanilla and milk. Add melted butter. Mix well. Pour over cherries. Bake 40-50 min. or until golden brown. Dust with powdered sugar or cream cheese glaze (see recipe) when cool.

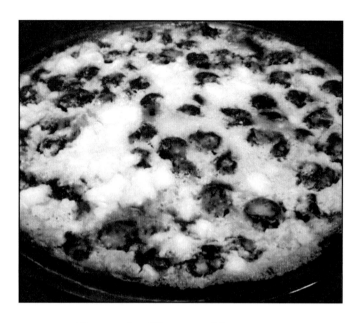

French Cherry Dessert

Prep Time: 25 min.

Cook Time: 40-50 min.

Makes: 8 servings

2 1/2 c cherries, pitted

2 Tbsp powdered sugar

3 eggs

1/2 c sugar

1/4 tsp salt

3/4 c all-purpose rice flour blend

1 tsp vanilla extract

1 c cream

2 Tbsp butter, melted

2 Tbsp cream cheese, softened

1. Preheat oven to 350°F. In greased 10-in. round cake pan or pie pan, layer in cherries. Sprinkle with powdered sugar.

2. In bowl, combine eggs, sugar, and salt. Whisk together. Add rice flour and beat until incorporated. Add vanilla, cream, melted butter, and cream cheese; mix well.

3. Pour over cherries. Bake 40-50 min. or until golden brown. Dust with powdered sugar or cream cheese glaze (see recipe) when cool.

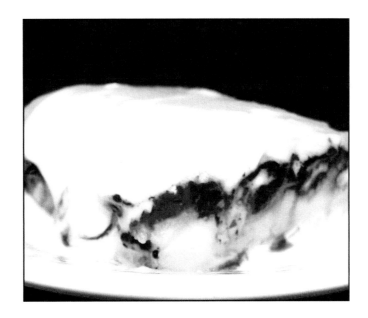

Blueberry Dessert

Prep Time: 25 min.
Cook Time: 40-50 min.
Makes: 8 servings

2/3 c sugar, divided

2 c blueberries

4 eggs

1/4 tsp salt

3/4 c all-purpose rice flour blend

1 tsp vanilla

1 c milk

2 Tbsp melted butter

1. Preheat oven to 350°F. Grease 10-in. round cake pan or 9x9 pan. Dust with 2 Tbsp sugar and layer in blueberries. In mixing bowl, add eggs, remaining sugar, and salt; whisk together. Add rice flour until incorporated. Stir in vanilla and milk.

2. Add melted butter. Mix well. Pour over blueberries. Bake 40-50 min. until golden brown. Dust with powdered sugar or cream cheese glaze (see recipe) when cool.

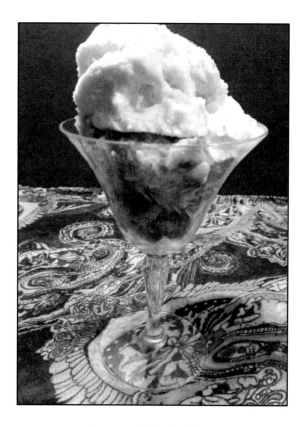

Bread Pudding

Prep Time: 20 min.
Cook Time: 1 hr.
Makes: 4-6 servings

4 c yeast bread cubes (p.179)

2 eggs

3/4 c milk

1/4 c cream

2 Tbsp sugar

1/4 tsp vanilla

dash salt

1. Preheat oven to 350°F. Place bread cubes in greased 9x9 pan. In bowl, mix together eggs, milk, cream, sugar, vanilla, and salt until smooth. Pour over bread cubes.

2. Press bread cubes to absorb the liquids. Cook 1 hr. until set and cooked through. Serve warm with ice cream.

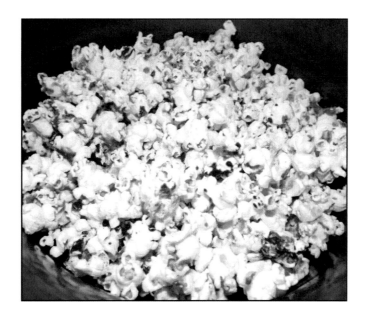

Caramel Corn

Prep Time: 5 min.

Cook Time: 6-10 min.

Makes: 10 servings

1/2 c dark or light corn syrup

3/4 c white or brown sugar

1/2 tsp salt

2 Tbsp butter

12 c popped popcorn

1. Preheat oven to 375°F. Mix syrup, sugar, salt, and butter in saucepan. Cook until mix starts to bubble, about 1 min.

2. Pour over popcorn and coat pieces. Place on greased cookie sheet. Bake 5 min., break apart into bowl and serve.

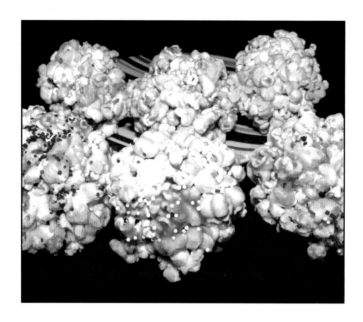

Popcorn Balls
Prep Time: 10 min.
Cook Time: 10 min.
Makes: 6-8 balls

3/4 c brown sugar
1/4 c honey
2 Tbsp butter
10-12 c popped popcorn

1. In saucepan, over low heat, combine brown sugar, honey, and butter. Stir occasionally until mixture bubbles around the edges.

2. Pour mixture over popcorn, stirring to coat. Grease hands lightly with butter and form popcorn into balls. Can add sugar sprinkles, food coloring, or flavored oils (cherry, mint, etc.) to balls to make more festive.

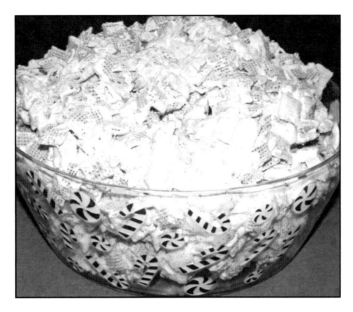

Sweet Party Mix

Prep Time: 5 min.

Cook Time: about 3 min.

Makes: I pan

3 Tbsp butter

I pkg (10 oz) marshmallows

I box (12-14 oz) rice or corn square cereal

1. Microwave butter in bowl until melted. Add marshmallows, coat with butter.

2. Microwave 45 sec, stir, then microwave 1 1/2 min. until marshmallows are melted.

3. Add cereal, mix well. Press into greased baking pan, add sugar sprinkles. Cool. Crumble apart before serving.

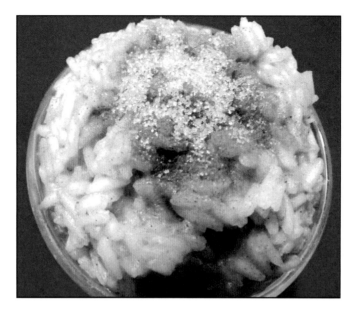

Sweet Rice

Cook Time: 17-23 min.

Makes: 2-4 servings

3 c water

1 c rice, uncooked

1/2 c milk

1 tsp cinnamon (optional)

1/2 c sugar

1. Boil water in a saucepan. Add rice and cook until tender and most of the water is gone, about 15-20 min.

2. Add milk, cinnamon, and sugar. Cook on high, stirring constantly until rice thickens again, about 2-3 min. If too thick, add more milk.

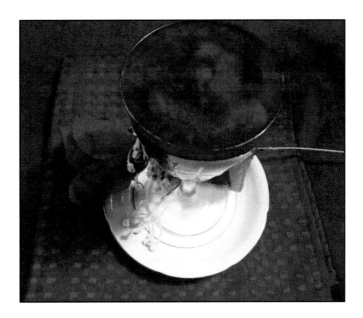

Fruit Soup

Prep Time: 10 min.
Cook Time: 15 min.
Makes: 5-6 cups

1 c apples, cored, peeled, and sliced
1 c pears, cored, peeled, and sliced
1 c strawberries, sliced
1 c red seedless grapes, cut in half
1 c blueberries
1 Tbsp sugar
1/2 c water
2 Tbsp cornstarch mixed in 1 c cold water

1. In saucepan, combine apples, pears, strawberries, grapes, blueberries, sugar, and water. Set on high and cover. Cook 5 min. until it starts to steam. Reduce heat to low and cook until apples are tender.

2. Return to high heat and add cornstarch mixture, cooking until it thickens. Serve hot. Good with vanilla ice cream or cold over yogurt.

Variations: Can use all or just some of the fruits listed. Can also use thawed frozen fruit in place of fresh.

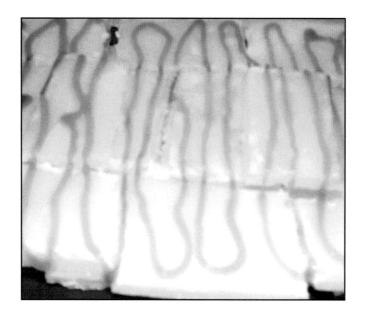

Butter Toffee

Prep Time: 5 min.
Cook Time: 10 min.
Chill Time: 2-3 hrs.
Makes: 1 pan

1/2 c unsalted butter, melted

1 c sugar

2 Tbsp water

1/2 tsp vanilla

1/4 tsp salt

1. In saucepan, add melted butter, sugar, water, vanilla, and salt together over medium heat. Let dissolve. Stir enough to have ingredients melt together, but not too much or it will get hard and sticky.

2. Spread on either greased cookie sheet or parchment paper. Cool completely to harden.

Variations: Can use salted butter and leave out the extra salt. Can add some rum flavoring as well.

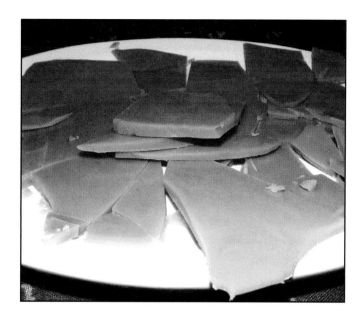

English Toffee

Prep Time: 5 min.
Cook Time: 12-15 min.
Makes: 1 pan

1 c sugar

2 Tbsp water

1 c butter, salted

1/2 tsp vanilla

1. In a saucepan, mix together sugar, water, and butter. Cook on high, stirring occasionally. When it starts to bubble, time it for about 8 min. and a candy thermometer reads between 250-275°F. Test a small piece in cold water. If it cracks in the mouth, it's done.

2. Add in vanilla, stirring quickly. Spread in a greased baking pan. Let it cool completely. Break apart and serve.

Variations: Can use rum flavoring as well.

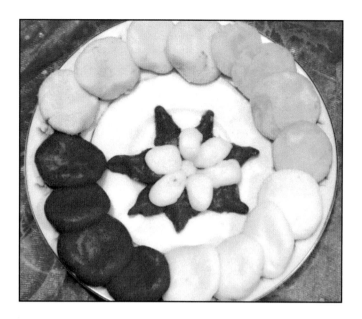

Cream Cheese Drops

Prep Time: 15 min.

Makes: about 36 pieces

3-oz cream cheese, softened

2 1/2 c powdered sugar

4 to 6 drops LorAnn Gourmet Flavoring

4 to 6 drops LorAnn Food Coloring

1. Mix cream cheese and powdered sugar together in bowl. Add flavoring and food color, starting with 4 drops and increasing as desired.

2. Roll into balls or desired shapes. Refrigerate until ready to serve.

Variations: Can divide into fourths and flavor with 1 drop of food coloring and 1 drop of flavoring for each ball.

Used by permission from LorAnn Gourmet Foods

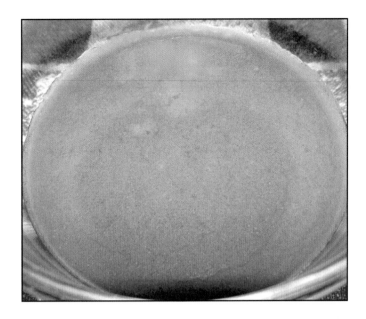

Caramel Sauce

Prep Time: 5 min.
Cook Time: 10-15 min.
Makes: 1/2 cup

1 Tbsp butter, salted
2 Tbsp brown sugar
1 tsp molasses
1/4 c whole milk or cream
1 tsp vanilla extract

1. In a saucepan, melt butter and brown sugar on high heat, stirring constantly. When lightly browned, add molasses and milk.

2. Cook until thickened. Add vanilla and cook about 1 min. more. Cool 5-10 min. and serve over ice cream or cake.

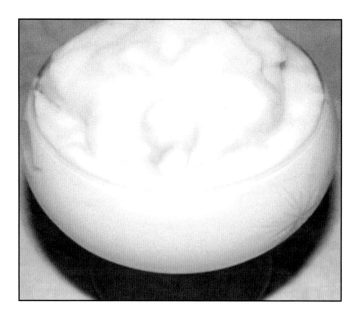

Custard

Prep Time: 5 min.
Cook Time: about 10 min.
Makes: 3 1/2 - 4 cups

1/3 c cornstarch

3 Tbsp sugar

2 Tbsp butter, salted

1 tsp vanilla extract

3 c milk

1. In bowl, combine cornstarch, sugar, butter, vanilla, and milk.

2. To cook in saucepan: add to saucepan. Cook on medium heat, stirring frequently, until thickened.

3. To cook in microwave: add to microwave-safe bowl. Cook high 4 min., then stir after every 2 min. Watch that it doesn't froth over. Keep adding 2 min. until thickened.

4. When cooled, it is common for a thin skin to form. Remove before serving.

Variations: Can add 1/2 tsp rum flavoring.

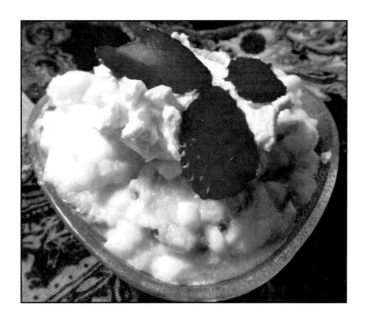

Strawberry Clouds

Prep Time: 10 min.

Makes: 4 cups

2 c cooked custard (p.170)

1 Tbsp milk

2 c sliced strawberries

1 c whipped cream (p.187)

1. In bowl, mix together the custard, milk, and strawberries. Spoon into serving dishes.

2. Top with whipped cream. Serve chilled.

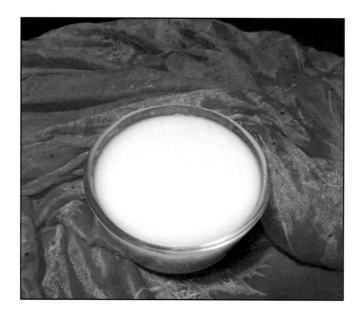

Vanilla Sauce

Prep Time: 10 min.
Cook Time: 3 - 5 min.
Makes: 1 1/2 cups

1/3 c sugar
1 Tbsp cornstarch
1/8 tsp salt
1 c cold water or milk
1 Tbsp butter
1 tsp vanilla extract

1. In saucepan, mix together sugar, cornstarch, and salt. Stir in cold water or milk. Cook on medium heat 3 - 5 min., stirring constantly until it thickens.

2. Remove from heat and add butter and vanilla. Stir until butter is melted.

Variations: Can use 1 c cold fruit juice for the liquid, such as apple or strawberry.

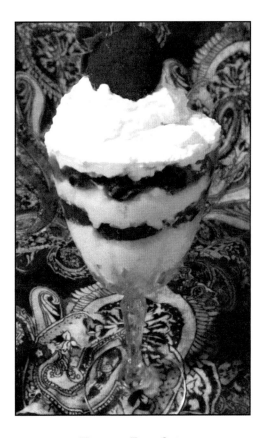

Fruit Parfait

Prep Time: 10 min.
Makes: 4 servings

1 c custard (p.170)

1/2 c strawberries, sliced

1 c plain yogurt

1/2 c blueberries

1/2 c whipped cream (p.187)

1. In serving glasses, layer custard on bottom layer. Add strawberries, then a layer of yogurt.

2. Next, add blueberries. Top with whipped cream. Serve chilled.

Variations: Can add different fruit if desired.

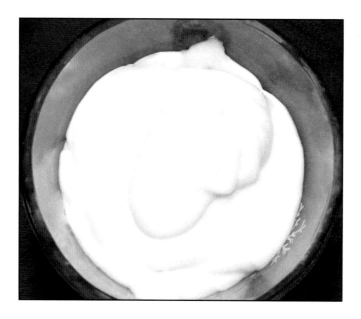

Cream Cheese Glaze

Prep Time: 5 min.

Makes: 1-2 cups

4 oz cream cheese, softened

1 Tbsp milk

2 c powdered sugar

1 tsp vanilla extract (optional)

1. In a bowl, mix together cream cheese, milk, and powdered sugar.

2. Blend until smooth. Can add 1 tsp vanilla extract for flavor if desired. Keep chilled.

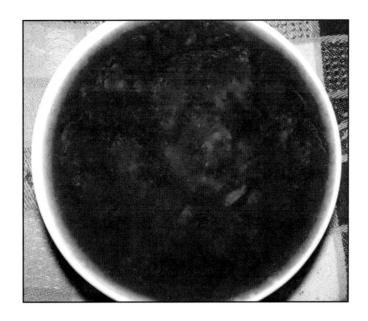

Slow Cooker Applesauce

Prep Time: 10 min.

Cook Time: 3-4 hrs.

Makes: 2-3 cups

4 c apples, peeled, cored, and sliced

1/2 c water

1 tsp cinnamon

1/2 c sugar

1. Add apples, water, cinnamon, and sugar to slow cooker, stirring to incorporate.

2. Turn on high for 2 hrs., then switch to low for 1-2 hrs. until apples are soft. Remove from slow cooker and whip with beater on medium until smooth. Eat warm or cold.

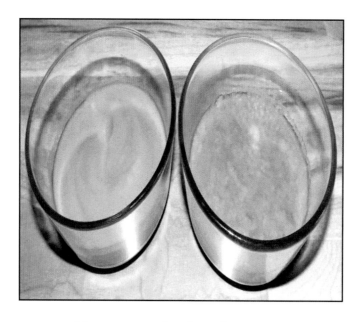

Homemade Applesauce

Prep Time: 15 min.
Cook Time: 15 min.
Makes: 2 cups

4 medium apples, peeled and sliced thin
1/2 cup water

1. Place apples in medium saucepan, add water.

2. Cover and cook on medium high heat, stir occasionally.

3. After 5 minutes, reduce heat to simmer. Cook 10 minutes or until apples are tender.

4. Mash or blend in food processor until smooth. May add sugar or cinnamon if desired.

Variations: Can use 4 cups frozen sliced apples. Cook for 10 minutes until tender.

Recipe can be doubled, add 5 minutes to cooking time.

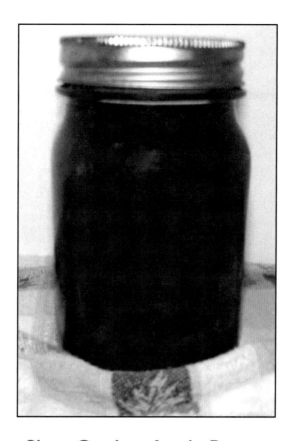

Slow Cooker Apple Butter

Prep Time: 15 min.
Cook Time: 2-3 hrs.
Makes: 3 cups

1/2 c sugar
1/2 c brown sugar
1 tsp cinnamon
1/4 tsp nutmeg
dash salt
1 tsp vanilla extract
4 c apples, peeled, cored, and sliced

1. In bowl, mix sugar, brown sugar, cinnamon, nutmeg, salt, and vanilla extract. Add apples, coating them with the sugars.

2. Add mixture to slow cooker. Turn on high 2 hrs., then turn down to low for 1-2 hrs. or until apples are soft. Place in bowl, blend with mixer on medium until smooth. Serve hot or cold, and can be stored in canning jars.

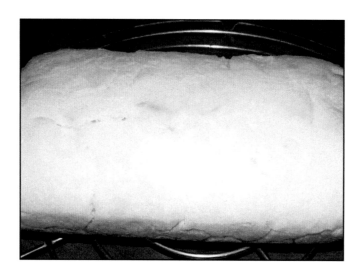

Yeast Bread

Prep Time: 15 min. plus 2-5 hrs. to raise

Cook Time: 40 min.

Makes: 1 loaf

1 Tbsp yeast

2 Tbsp sugar

1/2 c warm water

2 c all-purpose rice flour blend + extra to make less sticky

1 tsp salt

1/2 c lard (or butter)

1 c milk or warm water (between 105-110°F)

1. In small bowl, puff yeast by mixing yeast and sugar with water and letting it sit 5 min.

2. In large bowl, mix flour and salt. Cut in lard until crumbly. Add yeast mixture and milk; mix well. Add a little more flour to form a dough that's not too sticky.

3. Form into a loaf and place in greased bread pan. Let raise in a warm spot for about 2-5 hrs. Preheat oven to 350°F. Bake for 40 min. until golden brown.

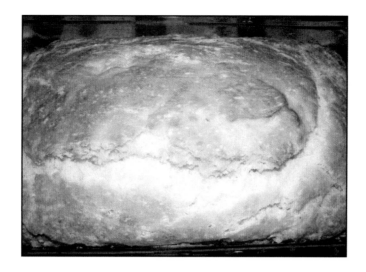

Irish Soda Bread

Prep Time: 15 min.
Cook Time: 60 min.
Makes: 1 loaf

2 c all-purpose rice flour blend

1/3 c white sugar

1 tsp salt

2 tsp baking soda

1/2 c butter

1 egg, beaten

1 1/2 c buttermilk

1 Tbsp vinegar

1. Preheat oven to 325°F. Combine flour, sugar, salt, and soda. Cut in butter.

2. In separate bowl, blend egg, buttermilk, and vinegar. Add liquid mixture to flour mixture.

Mix until moistened (don't over mix).

3. Pour mixture into greased loaf pan. Bake for 60 min. until golden and fluffy.

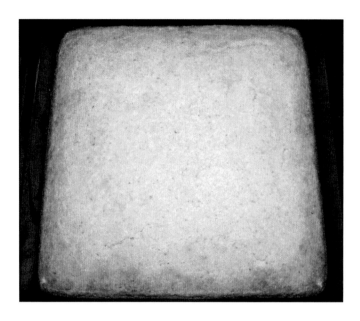

Golden Cornbread

Prep Time: 20 min.
Cook Time: 20-25 min.
Makes: 9 servings

1 1/4 c yellow cornmeal

1 c all-purpose rice flour blend

1/2 tsp salt

1/4 c sugar

1/2 c lard

1 egg

1 1/4 c milk

1 tsp apple cider vinegar

1. Preheat oven to 425°F. In bowl, mix together cornmeal, rice flour, salt, and sugar. Cut in lard.

2. In small bowl, whisk egg. Add milk and vinegar. Add to dry ingredients. Mix until moist.

3. Pour into greased 9x9 pan. Bake 20-25 min. or until center is cooked through.

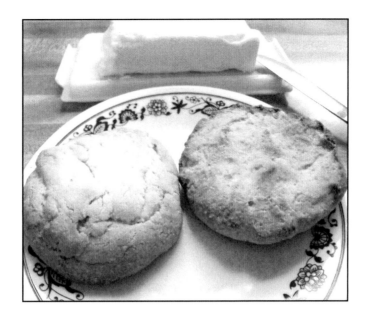

Johnny Cake Biscuits

Prep Time: 15 min.

Cook Time: 9-10 min.

Makes: 10-12 biscuits

1 1/4 c all-purpose rice flour blend

1 c white cornmeal

1 tsp baking soda

1/2 tsp salt

2 Tbsp sugar

1/2 c lard or butter

1/2 c milk mixed with 1 Tbsp white vinegar OR 1/2 c buttermilk (no vinegar)

1 egg

1. Preheat oven to 425°F. In bowl, mix rice flour, cornmeal, baking soda, salt, and sugar. Cut in lard until mixture is crumbly.

2. Add milk mixture, then egg. Blend until it forms a dough. Press into biscuit cutter on greased cookie sheet. Bake 9-10 min. or until golden.

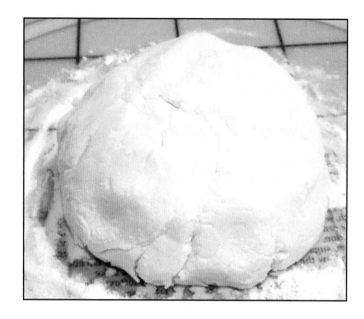

All-Purpose Rice Flour Dough

Prep Time: 10 min.

Makes: 1 dough

1 c all-purpose rice flour blend

2 eggs

dash salt

1/4 c water

1 Tbsp butter, softened

1. In bowl, mix together rice flour, eggs, salt, water, and butter. Add more water and flour as needed to create a dough that's not sticky.

2. Roll out on a floured surface and use as desired.

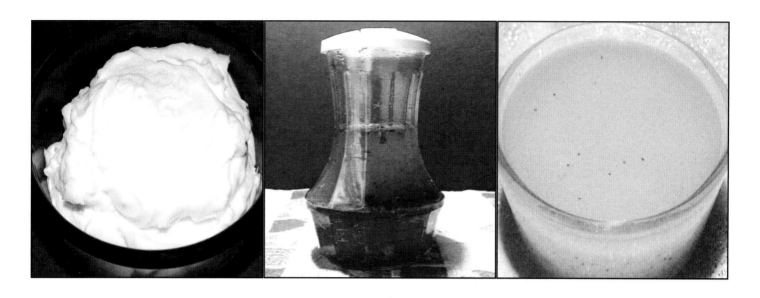

Quick Guide: Hints, Tips, & Substitutions

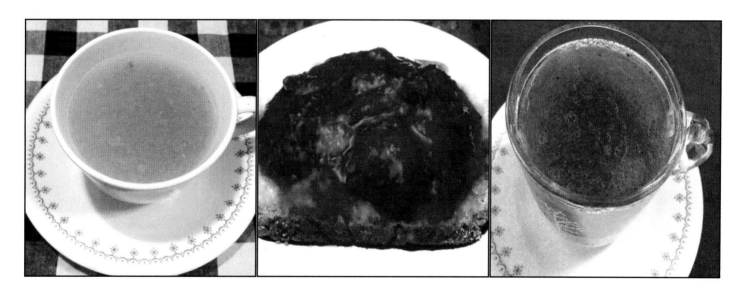

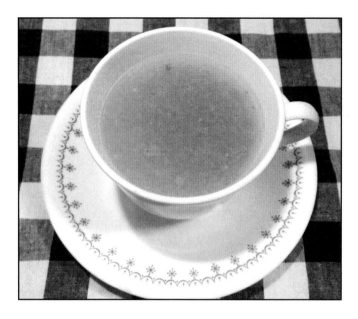

Chicken Broth

Prep Time: 5 min.

Cook Time: 2 hrs. 5 min.

Makes: about 8 cups broth

2-3 lbs chicken with bones, skinned

2 tsp salt

1 tsp black pepper

2 tsp seasoning salt

2 tsp onion powder

1/2 Tbsp celery salt or seed

8-10 cups water (enough to cover chicken)

1. In large stock pot, place chicken, salt, pepper, seasoning salt, onion powder, and celery salt. Cover with water. Heat on high for 5 min., then on low for 2 hrs.

2. Remove meat to use in a favorite recipe. Remove chicken bones and strain broth.

3. Can be refrigerated to be used right away, frozen to use later, or canned in jars to store for future use.

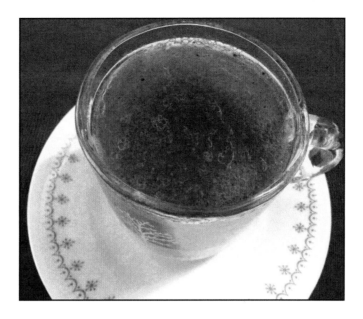

Beef Broth

Prep Time: 5 min.
Cook Time: 2 hrs. 20 min.
Makes: about 6 cups broth

1 Tbsp butter, salted

1 Tbsp olive oil

2-3 lbs. beef, whole or cubed without fat

2 tsp salt

1 tsp black pepper

2 tsp seasoning salt

2 tsp onion powder

8 cups water (enough to cover beef)

1. In a large stock pot, heat butter and olive oil. Add meat and brown on one side. Add salt, pepper, seasoning salt, and onion powder.

2. Add water to pot. Cook on high for 15 min. Reduce heat and cook on med-low heat for 2 hrs. Add more water if needed to cover meats. Remove meat to use in favorite recipe and strain the broth.

3. Can be refrigerated to be used right away, frozen for use later, or canned in jars to store for future use.

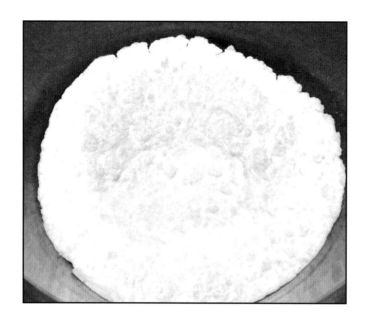

Baking Powder Substitute

Prep Time: 5 min.

Makes: 1 Tbsp

2 tsp cream of tartar

1 tsp baking soda

1/2 tsp salt

1. In bowl, mix together cream of tartar, baking soda, and salt. Combine until completely mixed.

2. Mix will not keep, so make each time you need it.

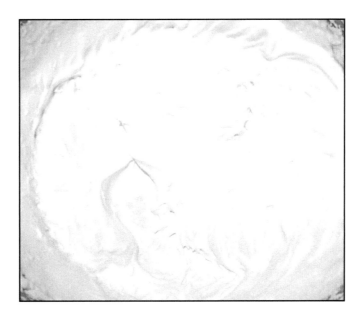

Whipped Cream

Prep Time: 2 min.

Makes: 1-2 cups

1 tray of ice cubes

1 c heavy whipping cream

2 Tbsp sugar

1 tsp vanilla extract

1. Place a smaller metal or glass bowl into a larger one. Add ice cubes between the bowl layers.

2. Add cream, sugar, and vanilla into smaller bowl. With electric beater, beat mixture on high until peaks form. Keep chilled.

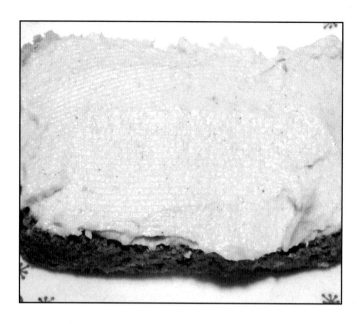

Honey Cinnamon Spread

Prep Time: 5 min.

Makes: 1 cup

1 pkg (8 oz) cream cheese, softened

2 Tbsp honey

1/2 Tbsp cinnamon

1/4 c powdered sugar

1. In bowl, blend together cream cheese, honey, and cinnamon. Add powdered sugar, blend.

2. Once smooth, place in container and keep chilled. Use on breads, pancakes, or as a sweet accent to cakes.

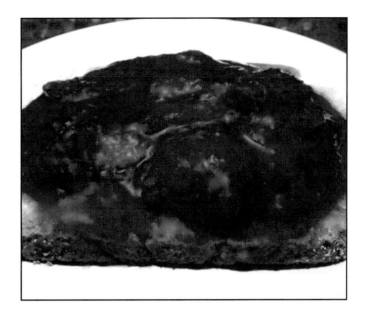

Strawberry Rhubarb Jam

Prep Time: 10 min.
Cook Time: 30 min.
Makes: 5 8-oz jars

3 c sugar

2 c frozen rhubarb, cut into 1/2-in. slices

4 c fresh or frozen strawberries, sliced

1. Combine sugar with rhubarb and strawberries in stock pot. Simmer 10 min., then bring to boil. Stir frequently until thickened, about 20 min.

2. Strain off froth. Can cool and keep in refrigerator or pour into canning jars and seal.

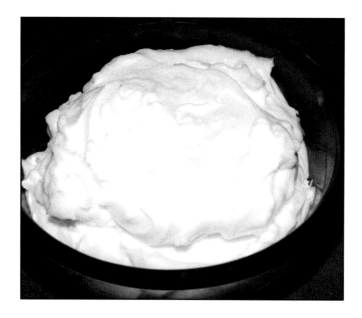

Homemade Mayonnaise

Prep Time: 5 min.

Cook Time: 5-10 min.

Makes: 4 cups

3/4 c canola oil or olive oil

1 1/2 tsp salt

1/4 tsp yellow mustard

2 beaten eggs mixed with water to make 3/4 c

2/3 c cornstarch mixed with 1 c cold water

2 Tbsp sugar

1/3 c white wine vinegar or distilled vinegar

1. Combine in blender canola oil, salt, mustard, and egg mixture. Blend until smooth.

2. In saucepan, cook together cornstarch mixture, sugar, and vinegar until stiff. While hot, add to blender mixture and blend smooth.

3. Refrigerate and use in cooking or on bread. Will keep for about 1 month.

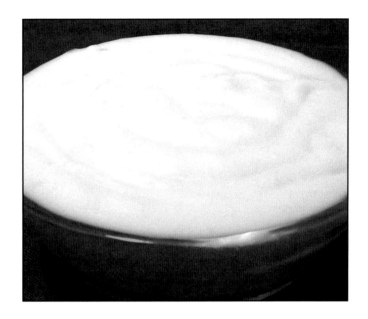

Homemade Salad Dressing

Prep Time: 5 min.

Cook Time: 5-10 min.

Makes: 4 cups

3/4 c canola oil or olive oil

1 1/2 tsp salt

1/4 tsp yellow mustard

1 egg beaten mixed with water to make 3/4 c

2/3 c cornstarch mixed with 1 c cold water

1/2 c sugar

1/3 c distilled vinegar

1. Combine in blender canola oil, salt, mustard, and egg mixture. Blend until smooth.

2. In saucepan, cook together cornstarch mixture, sugar, and vinegar until stiff. While hot, add to blender mixture and blend smooth.

3. Refrigerate and use in cooking or on bread. Will keep for about 1 month.

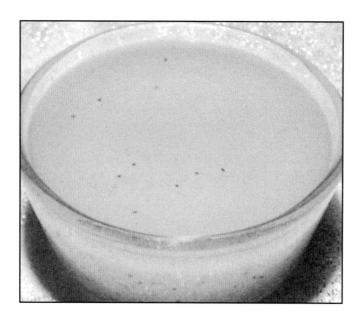

Sweet Onion Dressing

Prep Time: 5 min.

Makes: 1 1/2 - 2 cups

1 c canola oil

1/4 c vinegar or white wine vinegar

1/2 c sugar

1 small onion, chopped

1/2 tsp celery seed

1/4 tsp yellow mustard

1 tsp salt

1. In blender, mix together canola oil, vinegar, sugar, onions, celery seed, mustard, and salt.

2. Refrigerate or use in cooking. Keep cold.

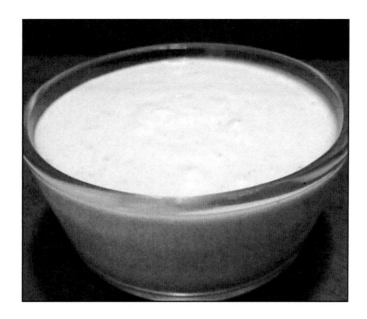

Thousand Island Dressing

Prep Time: 5 min.

Makes: about 1 cup

2 Tbsp ketchup

1 Tbsp white vinegar

2 tsp sugar

1 Tbsp sweet pickle relish

1/8 tsp salt

1/2 c mayonnaise

1. In bowl, combine ketchup, vinegar, sugar, relish, salt, and mayonnaise. Stir well.

2. Place dressing in a covered container and refrigerate. Keep cold.

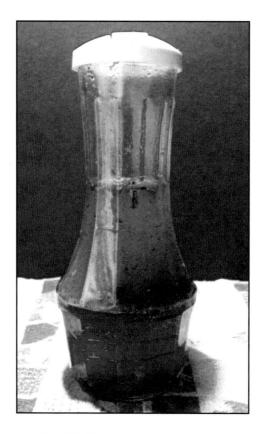

Red Wine Vinaigrette

Prep Time: 5 min.

Makes: 1-2 cups

1/2 c olive oil

1/2 tsp black pepper

1 1/2 tsp Italian seasoning

1 tsp salt

1/2 tsp sugar

2/3 c red wine vinegar

1. In bowl, combine olive oil, pepper, Italian seasoning, salt, sugar, and red wine vinegar.

2. Place in a jar or container and shake well before using.

Important Measurements and Terms

tsp = teaspoon   Tbsp = Tablespoon   c = cup
pkg = package   ml = milliliter   oz = ounce

Conversions

cup	fluid oz	Tbsp	tsp	milliliter
1 c	8 oz	16 Tbsp	48 tsp	237 ml
3/4 c	6 oz	12 Tbsp	36 tsp	177 ml
2/3 c	5 oz	11 Tbsp	32 tsp	158 ml
1/2 c	4 oz	8 Tbsp	24 tsp	118 ml
1/3 c	3 oz	5 Tbsp	16 tsp	79 ml
1/4 c	2 oz	4 Tbsp	12 tsp	59 ml
1/8 c	1 oz	2 Tbsp	6 tsp	30 ml
1/16 c	.5 oz	1 Tbsp	3 tsp	15 ml

Index

Manufactured by Amazon.ca
Bolton, ON

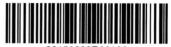